Sarah Vincent knew she wanted to be a writer when she was ten. She was a playwright for fifteen years, then turned to writing books. *Death by Dim Sim* is her tale of her battle with her weight and finally losing 40 kilos. She is currently working on her detective novel *The Fake Detective* and several picture books. She lives with her husband and two children, plus a very bossy cat and a dog that loves to lick everything.

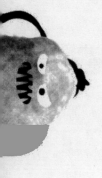

DEATH BY DIM SIM

A MEMOIR

HOW I BEAT OBESITY

SARAH VINCENT

WILLIAM HEINEMANN: AUSTRALIA

*Advice is of a general nature only and people should consult their own
doctor or health practitioner before following any of the health, exercise
and dietary advice offered here.*

A William Heinemann book
Published by Penguin Random House Australia Pty Ltd
Level 3, 100 Pacific Highway, North Sydney NSW 2060
www.penguin.com.au

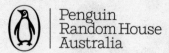

Penguin
Random House
Australia

First published by William Heinemann in 2017

Addresses for the Penguin Random House group of companies can be found at
global.penguinrandomhouse.com/offices.

National Library of Australia
Cataloguing-in-Publication entry

Vincent, Sarah, author
Death by Dim Sim/Sarah Vincent

ISBN 978 0 14378 211 7 (paperback)

Vincent, Sarah
Weight loss – Anecdotes
Low-carbohydrate diet
Low-carbohydrate diet – Recipes
Reducing diets
Fat
Natural foods

Front cover illustration by FenrisWolf, courtesy of Shutterstock
Back cover images by Liskus, courtesy of Shutterstock
Cover design by Adam Laszczuk
Internal design by Midland Typesetters, Australia
Typeset in 12/16.5pt Berkeley LT by Midland Typesetters, Australia
Printed in Australia by Griffin Press, an accredited ISO AS/NZS 14001:2004 Environmental
Management System printer

Penguin Random House Australia uses papers that are natural, renewable and recyclable
products and made from wood grown in sustainable forests. The logging and manufacturing
processes are expected to conform to the environmental regulations of the country of origin.

To Russell,
I love you fiercely

Contents

Part One

How I freed myself from my prison of fat

Chapter One

122 kilos

I've worked at a desk most of my life. Making calls and answering emails. But at three o'clock each afternoon I would answer a very special call – the call of the dim sim. If you don't know what a dim sim is – perhaps because you've never bought food cooked in ten-day-old oil and served with enough salt to preserve an elephant – let me explain. Dim sims are an Australian invention; a fusion of Asian and Australian tastes, but not in a cutting-edge, inner-city kind of way. It's a scoop of meat (beef, pork, chicken, horse?) mixed with random vegetable ends (cabbage, carrot, turnip?), shaped into a hand grenade, wrapped in pastry, deep fried and then, for extra goodness, drowned in soy sauce. They were invented in Melbourne, my home town, in the 1920s. Cheap, filling and quick, they soon became a favourite of the working class, an ever-present item in every takeaway shop in the country. One dim sim will set you back about a dollar, and a bag of three was my occasional budget-friendly way to beat my afternoon energy slump.

But working for several years in a particularly stressful job with a huge workload, my occasional treat became a daily regime and my weight crept from 95 to 122 kilos. Already seriously overweight, I became morbidly obese. My office was in the rear of a hospital – so in the rear it was in a metal portable in the car park. At three o'clock each afternoon I'd thread my way through the parked cars to the hospital cafeteria where a lovely display of fried goodies waited. There was healthy food there too, but alfalfa doesn't quite call to me like grease and salt do.

On my way through the cars I had to run the gauntlet of patients who had come out for a smoke. Smoking was banned on hospital grounds, so on crutches or in wheelchairs, and dragging their IV poles, they would line up along the car park fence to get their nicotine fix. Summer or winter, rain or heatwave, they would be there in their pyjamas. They were not a cheery bunch. There was no chatting or camaraderie. Always pale and gaunt, and sometimes missing a limb, they would stay for five minutes then shuffle back to their ward.

I'm not a smoker and would pass them inwardly shaking my head in disbelief. Didn't they realise they were probably in hospital because of their smoking-related disease? Wasn't being in hospital enough of a wake-up call to quit? Then one momentous day, as I passed them wrapped in smug self-righteousness, I had an epiphany, and not a pleasant one. Off to get my daily dimmies I realised I was just like them. If they were doing 'death by cigarette', then surely I was doing 'death by dim sim'. The only real difference between them and me was that I wasn't wearing pyjamas, and the only thing I could feel good about was that I still had time to do something about my addiction. If I wanted to see my kids grow up. If I wanted to live.

So, I stopped eating dim sims and biscuits and ice-creams and all the other foods I knew were bad for me and began to eat fresh wholesome food in moderation and to exercise regularly . . .

Are you kidding? Of course I didn't.

I did what I'd done since I first developed a weight problem when I was thirteen: I went on a crash diet. This one was a fruit diet. Fruit and nothing else. Watermelon mostly, plus oranges and apples, with my big treat for the day being a banana. I spent each day dreaming about that one banana. It was like a weight loss/detox/health trip all rolled into one. I felt light-headed most of the time and hungry all of the time. And boy did I pee a lot. I lasted a week. It was spaghetti carbonara that broke me. So creamy and bacony. The small amount of weight I did lose came straight back on before I could say, 'Pass the garlic bread.'

This had been pretty much the pattern all my life. I was either dieting and fighting constant food cravings, or giving in to the cravings and mindlessly eating everything in sight. I didn't really know how to eat normally. I didn't even know what normal was.

But this time I was determined to conquer my greed and gluttony and sloth. I climbed on the Garcinia Cambogia band-wagon. Oprah's doctor said it worked. It had 95 per cent HCA, whatever that is. Plus, it was an ancient fruit extract from Indo-nesia. Indonesia! And it was a fruit! It must be the answer.

It wasn't.

Then I bought a $500 gym membership. I went twice. Twice! That's $250 per visit. You would think for that amount they would have rolled out the red carpet and put me on gold-plated workout machines. But there was no carpet or gold-plated anything. Just me wasting more money.

In desperation I got my husband to take a photo of me in my underwear and put it on the fridge so I had to look at it every time I opened the door. I took it down the next day when a friend dropped by. No one needed to see me in my underwear. I certainly didn't want to. As soon as she left I went to the bookshop and bought a book on eating mindfully. I read it from cover to cover and followed all its suggestions about eating calmly and awarely. I ate calmly and awarely all day long and then mindlessly ate chocolate biscuits in bed at night.

It was the same old, same old. Get excited about the latest fad, convince myself that I had finally found the answer, tell everyone I was absolutely committed this time to losing weight and getting fit, then failing miserably and putting any weight I did lose straight back on, and then some. I'd do any celebrity gimmick, new fad or sign-your-wallet-away program. Packaged food delivered to your door? You betcha! Cabbage soup? Sure thing! Eat according to your blood type? Book me in!

And manic exercise programs? I did them too. Celebrity videos, too many gym memberships to count and even a 6am boot camp run by a South African army sergeant who told me I disgusted him. I would slavishly devote myself to each new diet and exercise regime, battling hunger and brain fuzz and low energy until I couldn't fight them anymore and gave in to chocolate and pasta and, of course, dim sims.

It was not until two years after my car park epiphany and many more crash diets that I decided it was time to do something sensible, slow and long term. I knew this time had to be different, because one of my beloved and very overweight uncles had just been diagnosed with advanced bowel cancer that had spread to his liver. He was doing well, but his diagnosis was a reminder that I needed to take care of myself – after all, I'd had the family curse five years before. I had been diagnosed with bowel cancer when I was forty-one, when my kids were five and one, and although I was lucky that it was caught early, I knew my excess weight and lack of exercise were greatly increasing the risk of it returning, and making me a target for other serious health problems.

So, I threw out the pills and the potions and joined Weight Watchers. I went to my first meeting and stood on their scales. My scales at home were broken (from overstrain, I fear), so I didn't know exactly what I weighed. I looked down and saw that my decision to take this level-headed approach was vindicated. The Weight Watchers scales showed that despite all the time, effort and money I had spent on fads since the epiphany, I had dropped only 4 kilos. I was 118 kilos. I was done with gimmicks forever.

The lady running the group saw that I was a newbie and sat me down for a chat. I told her about my goals and my long history of yo-yo dieting. She understood. She had been there herself. She said she had finally lost weight through Weight Watchers and was now teaching others to do the same. She talked me through the points program and said to be gentle on myself the first week. It was a lot to get used to and even a small loss would be an achievement, she said. She also outlined how successful weight loss was about long-term commitment rather than intense short bursts that would always fizzle out. The most important thing, she said, was to stick to the program, get back on it if I fell off and keep coming to meetings.

I knew she was right. I was there for the slow, sensible approach. But nonetheless part of me wanted to lie on the floor kicking my feet like a toddler and shouting, 'Where's the rare plant from Brazil that I brew into a tea and drink ten times a day? Don't you know how lazy and hopeless I am? I want the miracle!'

I resisted the urge. I took away her brochures and got started straightaway. And just like she said, it was a hard week. It wasn't a crash diet but it was a diet. And like all diets, I was hungry and grumpy all the time and I thought about food even more than

I usually did. And the brain fuzz was bad, especially in the after-noons, and my tiredness was off the scale. I had always struggled a lot with brain fuzz and low energy. I would wake up tired and go to bed tired and in between I was, pretty much, well, tired, which wasn't helpful for a middle-aged mum with two kids, working part-time and studying part-time. But now I couldn't reach for my high-sugar, high-carb foods to give me a quick energy boost.

I wrote down everything I ate – which was something I hated doing (first rule of crime: hide the evidence) – and returned a week later. To be honest I hadn't stuck 100 per cent to the plan, so I was a bit disappointed in myself, but I was also proud that I was back to learn more and to keep going. I put my food diary on the table in front of her and got on her scales. She looked at my very small weight loss, peered at my diary, wagged her finger and tsk-tsked me in front of the whole group. Then she called out, 'Next.'

What? Where was the lovely, go-slow-you'll-get-there lady from last week? Did she have an evil twin? Was last week's lady locked in a cupboard while her double humiliated me in public? I sat through the meeting downhearted, waiting for Nice Twin to come and find me and tell me I'd done okay, but she didn't appear. Evil Twin gave a group lecture on how great Weight Watchers pre-packaged foods were. That the points for an apple and a Weight Watchers Chocolate Mousse were the same but the mousse was much more 'yummy'. She said this licking her lips and rubbing her tummy like we were children. As soon as her sermon was over I left, throwing every one of her brochures in the bin the second I was out the door.

I was dejected but I wasn't going to give up. I was determined to lose weight and get healthy. Surfing the web one night I found Overeaters Anonymous. Their approach wasn't any sort of diet;

it was about accepting that you were addicted to food and needed the support and skills to change. This made sense to me, because surely the problem was in my head, and until I fixed that I would never be able to control what I put in my mouth.

It was deep winter the night I parked near a church hall and made my way inside. It was intensely cold in the meeting room and there was only one other person there. A slim woman, about fifty years old, behind a table of brochures and books. Over her head hung an embroidered sign that said: *God, grant me the serenity to accept the things I cannot change, the courage to change the things I can, and the wisdom to know the difference.*

Serenity? I wouldn't have known serenity if it had bitten me on my very large arse. Did they really have that here? How could I get some? I tried to catch the eye of the lady behind the display, but she was very busy arranging her brochures. People started drifting in, laughing and chatting and bringing Antarctic wind in with them.

When there were about fifteen people present, the lady with the brochures told us all to sit down at the large table. As she took her seat, busily getting the big minute-taking book ready, I looked around. There were a few youngsters and much older people at the table, but mainly there were women, like me, in their forties. I mentally tallied everyone's size: some were slim and some were middling. I wasn't one of the largest there, but I was close. Measuring my weight against other people was something I used to do constantly. In a meeting, on a train, at a party – I'd line everyone up on an invisible scale to see where I fitted in. It wasn't about judging others; it was about trying to figure out a sense of my own size. You see, most of the time I couldn't picture how I looked. My shape was blurry. I'd shrunk and grown so many times over the years I didn't know where I started and where I stopped.

9

When Brochure Lady had her notes in order she led us in the serenity prayer from the wall hanging and then announced, looking at me, that any new members present shouldn't hold up the meeting by sharing. That it was best they just sat and listened for their first few visits. She then handed over to the member who was running that night's meeting. That member, a girl in her twenties, smiled at me and said we would start, as usual, by going round the table and everyone would say their first name and how their week had been.

When it came to my turn I just said my first name. Nothing else, as instructed. Everyone else described in detail what a lousy week they'd had. How they had broken their eating plan and how angry and disappointed they were. Then a young girl who had just quit her job at a chocolate factory (good move) read from a big book, Brochure Lady gave a closing promise and appointed a different member to run the next meeting, and it was over. A piece of paper was passed around for those who wanted to provide their names and phone numbers to call each other for support. I added my name and number to the list.

Everyone left in chatty, jolly groups and Brochure Lady went back to her display. I timidly approached her and asked how I should get started and what I should do next.

'Just keep coming to meetings.'

'Is there anything else I should be doing?'

She sighed, snatched up a few of her brochures and flicked them at me. I took them and left.

I went back twice. Brochure Lady never got any friendlier and I never figured out what I was supposed to do, despite reading some of her books and listening to numerous podcasts. I was never offered a sponsor, I never shared my story and no one ever phoned me to offer support. And every week, without fail, I listened to fifteen or so people describe how they had binged on food that week. There was never one who said, 'I had a great week, this is really working for me.' Not one tiny chink of serenity ever peaked through anyone's dark cloud.

So, I never gave my will over to a higher power or humbly asked him to remove my shortcomings, as the twelve steps laid out. After three meetings I figured this higher power had better things to do than help a fat woman in the suburbs stop eating herself to death. He sure as hell wasn't helping anyone in that freezing church hall.

But I wasn't quite done trying. Still thinking the problem was all in my head, I next tried a hypnotherapist. She was a very nice woman who mostly worked with smokers but had helped a few people to lose weight. I lay on her comfy couch as she talked calmly to me. She placed the thought in my head of picturing an apple every time I felt like eating chocolate or chips or dim sims or anything else unhealthy. It worked. I love apples. Every time I craved bad food the image of a juicy Red Delicious would appear in my mind. And then I would eat the bad food anyway, followed by an apple. We went through a lot of apples at our house but I didn't lose any weight.

Still refusing to give up, I saw an ad for a doctor who had a new approach to weight loss. First thing Monday morning I phoned for an appointment. He was so busy he couldn't see me for three weeks. I booked in and waited impatiently, hoping he had the answer.

His office was in a leafy well-to-do suburb. He didn't have a receptionist, it was just him. He talked me through his program and showed me an online video. He seemed bored as he gave me the URL and my password and outlined how and when I needed to watch the video. Then he got me to sign two Medicare slips –

11

all above board, he promised, just a way to help him bulk-bill his clients. Three seems to be my magic number for giving things a go. I saw him three times over several weeks and watched his video every day. It didn't work.

During those weeks I kept thinking that if he really had the solution to successful weight loss, why did he seem so bored? And why didn't he have any testimonials from grateful clients on his wall? And the big question: if his program was so successful, why did he (I suspected) need to commit Medicare fraud to keep it going?

Then I decided that the problem wasn't in my head, that I just needed to eat less and move more. I hired an exercise bike for six months. I rode it several times, then hung washing from it to dry.

And then I gave up. Totally, completely, utterly. I was just too fat, too lazy, too greedy, too useless, too hopeless. No one had the answer. Not Weight Watchers, nor Overeaters Anonymous, nor the hypnotist, nor the dodgy doctor. I figured I may as well enjoy my chocolate and dim sims and sit on the couch watching TV with my husband every night and not bother anymore. I'd tried slow and sensible and it hadn't worked. I'd tried fixing my head and it hadn't worked either. I resigned myself to being fat for the rest of my possibly very short life.

And then I lost my stressful job. I didn't lose it as in I-put-it-down-somewhere-and-forgot-where-it-was; my contract wasn't renewed. I'd given my all to that job. I was devastated.

My husband, Russell, suggested I take some time off. Our youngest was starting primary school in seven months. 'Why not spend some time at home with her, then get her settled into school,' he said. 'Then look for a less stressful job. Get your smile back.'

What an amazing, supportive man. I agreed, suddenly looking forward to the months ahead; it had been so long since I had looked forward to anything. Luckily we were in the fortunate situation of having some money in the bank, for once. At about the time Russell and I started dating I had bought a house. This was before the property boom when a single person with $8000 in savings could buy property. Instead of buying a nice tidy flat, which would have been sensible, I'd bought a 1950s house that was sloping so badly to one side it looked like it was smiling. I lived there until we found out I was pregnant a year and a half later. That night I moved into Russell's house, just for a few days, and never left. Russell renovated my sloping house and then we rented it out to a lovely family. We hung on to it till we could no longer manage the loss we were making on it every year and thought the property boom was about to bust. I had been wrong about the boom ending but it did mean we had a nest egg when we sold it.

So, I spent six weeks sleeping in and catching up with friends. I refocused on my studies, getting my assignments done well in advance instead of the night before. I sat in cafes and read the paper. I had a massage. I kicked a footy with our son after school. I picked our daughter up from preschool and we went and had our nails done instead of my having to leave her with a friend and race off to work. We played board games together after dinner. We did craft. We went for long walks. It was bliss. And I had six and a half months left before my daughter started school and I needed to find another job.

And then Russell was diagnosed with cancer.

Chapter Two

118 kilos

Seriously? I'd had cancer five years ago and now Russell had it? Our kids were ten and six and *both* their parents had been diagnosed with cancer. Where was the justice in that? I wanted a second opinion. This was completely and totally wrong.

But it wasn't. It was cancer. Mine had been primary and hadn't spread. My surgeon had come rushing into my hospital room to give me the pathology from my operation with a big smile on his face. 'Best-case scenario,' he had said, beaming. Russell's oncologist wasn't beaming about his cancer. It was secondary and spreading. It was very, very serious.

After I told Russell the lump in his groin was a secondary cancer – yes, I had to tell him because he doesn't have a mobile phone, so his surgeon had to call me – I sat down on the lawn in our backyard and phoned my sister Ruth and wept.

'What will I do if he dies?' I asked her.

She didn't have an answer. What do you say to that?

Russell is possibly the best husband ever on the planet. I may have got in the wrong line when they were handing out waist-lines, but I was front and centre in the fabulous-husband queue. He's kind, funny, clever, caring, a great dad, handsome and did I mention kind? He is also a talented musician and a great cook, a trained masseuse and a children's librarian. And now he had a skin cancer on his torso that had spread to a lymph node in his right thigh.

As if that wasn't stressful enough, life was about to get even more complex. Russell is also a trained homeopath. Three weeks later, after he had finished all his tests and was due to have surgery – the only cure for this type of cancer – he cancelled the surgery and announced that he was treating himself with homeopathies and meditation.

I support natural therapies but I was very unsure about this. It was his life and his choice and he was 100 per cent sure he was doing the right thing, but we had two young children. Plus, all the doctors at the hospital were telling him that surgery as soon as possible was the only way to stop the cancer spreading from his lymph system to his brain or his lungs.

I didn't know what to do. Should I stop him? Should I support him? If his approach was going to work he needed my help. I was so confused and scared. In the end he was adamant, so I supported him the best way I could: by looking after the kids and giving him the room to undertake his meditation and his therapies.

And how did I support myself through the next few months? I ate. And boy did I eat. If I was an eating machine before his cancer, I became a monster-truck, all-consuming engine after his diagnosis. Every time I went to our local supermar-ket, which was daily, I was surprised there was anything left on the shelves from my previous visit. On top of eating huge meals and countless snacks, I was going to bed each night with a large block of chocolate and a whole packet of Tim Tam biscuits. That's eleven biscuits in case you're wondering. And I didn't care.

Having cancer yourself is hard. Watching someone you love have it is harder. Standing by while they refuse treatment and deal with it 'naturally' is stressful beyond belief. I wasn't angry with him; I was too dazed to feel much of anything. It felt like my head would explode if I tried to make sense of it all or think about what was going to happen.

These were the things I was trying not to think about: Should I tell him he had to have the surgery? Should I stop driving him to see all the natural therapy 'gurus' who thought what he was doing was great? Should I stop protecting him from the anger towards him felt by many people around us?

One decision I did manage to make, with the support of our amazing friend Lisa, who also happened to be an oncologist, was to get him and the hospital to work together to monitor his cancer regularly. And each scan showed that the cancerous lymph node was growing bigger.

After several months of staying calm and supporting him as best I could I needed to get away. I blew $300 of our savings on a fancy hotel room. I took our two kids and the three of us went and wore fluffy bathrobes and watched movies and splashed about in the room's huge bubbly spa bath, many miles away from the mess that was our home. If the kids hadn't fought with each other the whole time it would have been heaven.

Even though it wasn't the delightful getaway I'd hoped for, it did give me a break from Russell, which I desperately needed. When I got back I discovered he had spent the entire time we were away doing even more intensive meditation. Whoever said full-on meditation was good for you lied. He was so engrossed in it that he didn't speak to me or the kids or even acknowledge us when we got back. When he finally came out of his meditation room I told the kids to watch TV and took him out to the back garden and let him have it.

'Stop this shit and have the surgery or I'm leaving you and taking the kids.'

'No, Sarah, it's fine. It's great. I'm curing the cancer.'

'You're not curing the cancer. It's spreading. Do you not understand that?'

'I just need more time.'

'You don't fucking have more time!'

As I stomped inside I found my son standing in the shadow of the open back door. He'd heard every word.

'Are you leaving Dad?'

I tried to assure him that everything would be okay, that Daddy and I would sort it out, but he didn't listen. He just jumped on his bike and rode off.

I went into the kitchen, sat at the table and lay my head on the cool Formica. Would Russell have the surgery? Or would I have to follow through with my threat to leave and take the kids with me? How much would we get if we sold the house and split the money in two? Would it be enough for me and the kids to survive on? Would he die? And dear God why did our son have to hear what I'd just said?

Russell came in and sat next to me. 'I'm really scared, Sarah.'

I didn't lift my head. I couldn't look at him. I answered into the sleeve of my jacket. 'Good. I'm scared too.'

'No. You don't understand. I'm really scared. I'm hearing voices.'

This is when our lives stopped. On a Friday afternoon in April.

I called one of my sisters, Ruth, who is a nurse. She said to call the local Crisis Assessment and Treatment team straightaway. I did, and the CAT team came over an hour later.

My husband told the two psych nurses that he had been hearing voices for a month. I watched him talk to them, seeing him through their eyes; unshaven, telling them about frequencies and energies, about his obsessive homeopathic pills and how he could only eat foods that had the right vibrations.

You'd think I would have been filled with compassion, realising that he was so mentally unwell. But I became even more furious with him for dragging us all further down into this never-ending pit of misery. The lid on my anger had blown off and I couldn't get it back on. As the nurses tried to get him to describe what had been happening to him, I snarled at everything he said to them and pointed out that he had brought this all on himself with his stupid meditation and all the whackos he'd been seeing. The two CAT nurses kept telling me my anger wasn't helping him. They outlined the plan: they would visit every day and come back tomorrow with a psychiatrist to assess Russell and put him on medication. They asked me if I could cope with that. 'Sure thing,' I told them. We were already in hell, dropping down another level didn't make much difference and I was glad of the support.

As promised, the nurses came back the next day and brought a psychiatrist who took my husband's history, diagnosed psychosis brought on by severe stress, and prescribed anti-psychotic medication.

I told the kids the nurses were from the cancer hospital and kept them in the lounge room the whole time, watching TV so they didn't hear anything that was said. After the CAT team left I got them both bathed and into bed.

'Are you leaving Dad?' my son asked again as I read him a story.

'No, I was just mad at him,' I told him.

'Good, because I'm not going with you. I'm staying with Dad. He's nicer than you.'

He rolled over and crossed his arms.

I turned out his light. I didn't have an answer. How could I say, 'I know you love Dad but he's a mess and even though I'm not as fun as him I'm all you've got at the moment.' Instead I went to my bedroom, pulled out a new packet of double-coated Tim Tams and pushed them one after the other into my mouth. They're double-coated, so that was eight whole biscuits. By the final one I felt sick, but that was still better than feeling as if our lives were being smashed apart and that no amount of glue would ever put them back together again the same way.

The CAT team came every day. They would assess my husband and discuss his medication. I kept up the pretence that they were from the cancer hospital. Meanwhile Russell had found a new guru on the internet and was emailing him and talking to him on the phone daily.

I kept out of his way. Weeks passed.

And then something changed. My husband wasn't getting any better and I had to take him to the CAT team office to be reassessed. Every bad situation has a sliver of good. Even a wafer-thin sliver. The sliver of good in this one was that Psychiatrist Number Two convinced him to have the surgery. The psych nurses had all been pushing for it and so had I, but Psychiatrist Number Two got him over the line. I picked up the phone and booked Russell in before he changed his mind. I should have felt relief that finally the cancer would be removed, but all I felt was worry that he had left it too late.

Thankfully the operation went well and Russell was allowed to come home after a week. We had a 'Hospital in the Home' nurse visit to check his wound and his drain bag daily, as well as the CAT team every day and even another Psychiatrist, Number Three, who came to check his psychosis. Sometimes these visits happened all at the same time. Usually while the kids were at school, thank goodness. But all these visits didn't improve things. His surgical wound wasn't healing and neither was his head.

Russell was a grey ghost in slippers. He still had a drain bag and was losing fluid from the surgical site. He looked like he was developing an infection in the skin around the sutures. But these things could be fixed. Why was his head still such a mess? Why wasn't the medication for his psychosis working? How much longer could I pretend to the kids that he was just taking a lot of time to recover from the surgery? He wasn't saying or doing anything strange, he never did. If you spoke to him you would have thought he was perfectly normal – tired and listless, but perfectly normal. He just had this mess in his head he was trying to deal with all the time. He still played with the kids and chatted to friends when they came over. Only I could see the constant struggle he was having.

'I'm going to die,' he told me, exhausted one night, after I'd put the kids to bed.

'No, you're not,' I told him. 'The surgery went well. You're just healing slowly. The cancer nurses said that everyone is different. It'll come good. The drain bag will be out soon. The pathology from the surgery was good. The cancer was only in the one node. It hadn't spread to any others. You'll be fine.'

'No. I'm going to die. The voices are going to kill me. I have twenty-four hours to live.'

Luckily I had the CAT team on speed dial. They came over straightaway. The first question they asked was if he was really taking his medication. He admitted that he hadn't been. He'd been flushing his pills down the toilet all along because they made his psychosis worse.

One of the nurses sat with my husband in the lounge room while the other one took me into the kitchen. I had got to know them all pretty well over the past month. The nurse took my hand. 'I'm calling it, Sarah. Your husband has to be admitted. You can't manage this anymore and he needs to be in a psychiatric hospital. He can go of his own free will or we will call the police. If we call the police they will restrain him and put him in an ambulance. Either way, he is going. What do you think he will do?'

Just as it was me who had to tell Russell the cancer had spread, I opted to tell him that he needed to be admitted to a psychiatric hospital.

I quickly packed him a bag and promised to visit him every day. I phoned my other sister, Helen, and she dropped everything and came straight over to stay the night and look after the kids. I drove behind the two psych nurses as they took him to the large public hospital thirty minutes away that had a psych unit. He was put on a trolley in a cubicle in the Emergency department while we waited for a bed in the unit. We weren't allowed to pull the curtain across the front of the cubicle because he was a psych patient and had to be watched every minute. I talked softly to him and told him that everything would be okay. He didn't know what was real and what wasn't, so it didn't matter that I didn't sound very convincing.

After several hours in Emergency, he was visited by Psychiatrist Number Four, who took his history again and upped his medication. Then the psychiatrist took me aside.

'Does he choof?' he asked.

'Choof?' What did he mean? My husband wasn't a train.

I'd been in the Emergency department now for about seven hours and was very tired. Maybe he had said 'hoof', like a horse. But my husband wasn't a horse either.

'Hoof?' I asked.

'Choof? Smoke weed? Dope?' The psychiatrist mimed smoking a marijuana cigarette like he was in a Cheech and Chong movie.

'God no. We don't even drink alcohol. We watch TV.'

I don't think Psychiatrist Number Four believed me. I tried again. 'We really hate drugs. And we don't drink. Well, my husband has a beer on Christmas Eve with his brother-in-law. We really like TV, though. Period dramas and crime, but not gory crime. *Miss Fisher's Murder Mysteries*. We like Miss Fisher.'

I didn't find out if he liked Miss Fisher too. Another psych patient arrived, this time in handcuffs with a policeman on either side, and the doctor had to go. I went back to Russell as they settled the screaming man into the cubicle next to us. The agency nurse sitting at a desk constantly watching my husband now had someone more interesting to look at.

Then finally, three watching nurses and twenty-four hours later, my husband got a bed. I walked behind him as they wheeled him through a *Get Smart* series of security doors into the psych ward. A psych nurse came out from behind a floor-to-ceiling glass cage and showed us his room – it had two beds, separated by a toilet in the middle. The toilet had walls around it but no door; where there should have been a door there were saloon swing doors, like in a Western movie.

I didn't know any of the nurses here. And it was like no hospital I had ever been to. The nurse showed us around. Next to my husband's room was the rec room with some torn sofas and an old piano. She then showed us the art room, which had tables, some broken crayons (no pencils) and boxes and boxes of jigsaw puzzles, all with sticky notes on them saying there were missing pieces. There was a common area in front of the glass cage with a huge TV bolted to the wall with the volume on high. Watching it on more torn sofas was a group of blank-faced men and women who were also missing pieces.

It was now the next day, late evening, and Russell was very tired. We took him back to his room and Psychiatrist Number Five came and took his history (again) and upped his medication (again). Number Five couldn't tell us how long Russell would need to stay or if he would get any treatment. The nurse fetched his new dose of medication and stood over him while he took it. Clearly there would be no flushing it down the door-less toilet in this place.

I noticed there was no blanket on his bed and I asked the nurse for one. She went and looked but came back empty-handed. They were out of blankets. Then his roommate came into the room and went straight into the swing-door toilet and did the loudest bowel motion I have ever heard. Then someone started banging on the out-of-tune piano in the room next door. Then there was a code red and the nurse ran off.

It was at this point that I had to make the hardest decision of my life. How could I leave my husband here? How was he supposed to get better in this dangerous, cold, blanket-less place? How could I just abandon this man, whom I loved and who had nursed me through my own cancer?

But how could I take him home? I couldn't cope anymore and he wasn't getting better there. People think that I am the rock in our family. But I'm not. He's the one who keeps us all on track. He's the glue that makes our family work, and we needed him to get better.

I wondered if he would ever forgive me.

I walked past the staff who were pinning a screaming patient down on the floor as the sound of a police siren got closer. At the front security desk I told them I would be back to visit Russell in the morning. I asked again for a blanket. I left not knowing if he got it.

I told our kids their dad had gone to hospital because of an infection. I only told a few friends and family where he really was. When you have cancer people bring you casseroles. No one brings you casseroles when you have psychosis.

The next morning I woke up with a painful, puffy ankle, though I had no idea why. I asked Helen to take the kids to school and I drove myself to our small local hospital to make sure it wasn't serious. We didn't need anything else that was serious right now. The nurse and the doctor in Emergency made it very clear that I was a time-waster, and I felt their judgement as I hobbled over to the X-ray department in agony and sat there quietly waiting. It felt like the first quiet moment I'd had for a very long time. I let the busyness of the staff and patients swirl around me while I sat and thought about nothing.

Then my mobile rang. It was the psych unit. My husband was refusing to take his medication. I told them I'd be there soon.

I hung up and started sobbing. I hadn't cried since he'd first been diagnosed with cancer. I could hear that I was howling but I couldn't stop. I buried my head in my hands to try to muffle the noise, and I cried and cried and cried. I only stopped when I ran out of tears. The nurses in the X-ray department were nicer. They gave me tissues and a glass of water. I calmed down enough to have my X-ray and then they pushed me back to Emergency in a wheelchair and told me I had sprained my ankle. I was discharged and hobbled out to my car and set off for the psych hospital.

I visited Russell every day, and each visit he seemed exactly the same. He was taking his medication – they had told him they would section him if he didn't – but it wasn't helping him get better. At least a nurse from the main hospital was coming in every day to change the dressing on his wound and to check on his possible infection, so I didn't have to worry about that side of his recovery.

One morning I was just too tired to visit. After taking the children to school I phoned at 9.30 to get a message to him that I couldn't come. I asked the nurse who answered the phone what he was doing.

'Watching TV,' she told me.

My husband has never watched TV at 9.30 in the morning in his life. But what else do you do in that place? There was no treatment; it was just a holding pen until your medication kicked in. And his wasn't kicking in.

The next day he was due for a post-surgery check-up at the cancer hospital. When I picked him up and signed him out for the day, he seemed worse, even more vacant and bewildered. When I ran out of things to tell him about the kids or the house we continued the drive to the city in silence. At the cancer hospital, when his name was called, he needed my help to walk the twenty steps from the waiting room to the examination room. As soon as we got into the room I helped him to lie down on the bed as we waited for his doctor to arrive.

'Are you okay, hon?' I asked, feeling his forehead. He was cold and clammy. He shook his head.

'Are you sick? Are you coming down with something?'

He said his leg hurt. I helped him pull off his jeans so the doctor could see how he was recovering from the surgery. I'm no medical person but even I could tell there was something really wrong. There was a 20-centimetre circle of flaming red skin around his surgical incision.

25

'Wasn't a nurse from the main hospital coming in and dressing your wound every day?'

He looked at me with unfocused eyes. 'She never stayed long,' he said. 'I don't think she liked being in the psych unit.'

Clearly not. He was admitted back into the cancer hospital with a raging staph infection. Luckily, four days of intravenous antibiotics fixed it and it didn't get into his bloodstream or bones.

You know that sliver of good? We got it again. The psych team at the cancer hospital stepped in and took over his care. They changed his medication and in two days the voices were gone. I had my husband back and the kids had their father back.

When he was due to be discharged, one of the psychiatrists at the hospital took him on as a private patient and got him a room in a private psychiatric hospital thanks to $12,000 of our savings. I would spend it again in a heartbeat.

In this calm place with single rooms and blankets – such lovely fluffy blankets – and toilets with doors and where patients were under the care of one psychiatrist rather than five, he got better very quickly. There is a two-tier mental-health system in this country. The lower tier does have some wonderful people working in it but they are under-paid, under-staffed and totally under-resourced. They helped us out as best they could but we were lucky to be able to afford to be on the upper tier. It is a very different place on that top level. People actually get better up there – the people who can afford it.

After two weeks my husband came home and he completely recovered, physically and mentally, and our lives returned to normal. I even got a new job, working at Writers Victoria, an organisation that supports writers. My dream job, working with other writers and talking about writing all day long. My studies were going well again and Russell was back at work too. Life was back on track.

And our kids? How did we heal them? How do you put children back together after something like that? After my cancer we got a cat from the pound – a fluffy black bossy purring love-machine called Katman. Every evening when we went for a walk as a family Katman would try to come with us and we would have to pick him up and go back and lock him in the house. One night we decided to see how far he would follow us. Surely he would turn back? Nope. He followed us the whole way round the block, so the five of us started going for a walk each night.

This time we went to the pound to get a dog. When we got there we asked them if they had a medium-sized dog who liked kids and wasn't aggressive to other dogs or cats.

'You've just described the dog every family who comes here wants. If I had a hundred dogs like that I'd still need more,' the lady told us. But then she smiled. 'We do just happen to have one exactly like that today.' And she brought out a medium-sized leaping licking-machine called Lena.

On Lena's first day home she chased Katman through the house, thinking that because she was a dog and he was a cat and she was five times bigger she must be the boss. Katman soon put that misconception out of her head. Luckily both pets settled down quickly to a mostly happy system where Katman ruled the house and Lena ruled the backyard and whenever Lena stepped out of line Katman swiped her across the nose. Katman slept on my daughter's bed and Lena slept with her head on my son's pillow, wrapped in his arms. My son's nightmares vanished and he finally stopped asking me at bedtime each night if I was going to leave Daddy. All my assurances and apologies and explanations didn't help as much as a big goofy dog wriggling her way under his doona at lights out. My son forgave me and stopped worrying and when a story came on the radio about a famous person having cancer my daughter announced that cancer wasn't so bad – you just had surgery and then you were all better. There is nothing like pet therapy.

And my husband and me? Our marriage survived and, if anything, got stronger. My anger at him faded completely when I accepted and understood how scared, confused and mentally unwell he had been. His decision to cancel his surgery hadn't been made rationally, and that helped me comprehend his actions. Having cancer messes with your head. I certainly knew that. I'd needed a big dose of anti-anxiety medication and coun-selling after mine, and this wasn't my husband's first cancer. When he was twelve he'd had a sarcoma that had almost killed him. Another bullet he had dodged. Who knows what having cancer that young does to you?

I said before that no one brings you casseroles when you have psychosis. That's not exactly true. While we lost a few friends along the way, we were amazed by the number of friends and family who supported us, along with some wonderful neighbours and my husband's really caring work colleagues. I will never forget our friend Imogen bringing Russell flowers and sitting with him, or Andrea making a point of coming over to the car to talk to Russell when he was with me one day when I picked up the kids, or Terri offering to take our kids to the circus, or Rod and Bella visiting him in hospital.

There were so many slivers of good. The big sliver of good that came out of this whole situation (yes, there is one) is that whenever life gets overwhelming these days I think, *At least I'm not picking Russell up from a psychiatric hospital and driving him to a cancer hospital for a check-up.*

And now that life was getting back on track I got on a set of scales at my local shopping centre. I was 122 kilos. I stepped off and got on them again. Yep, 122. Despite all my over-eating I had only gained those same four pesky kilos back again. I realised something in that moment: 122 kilos was my set upper limit. No matter what I ate – and believe me, in the months Russell was sick I ate a lot – my body didn't seem able to go over 122. Perhaps it was a metabolism thing. Or perhaps my small amount of running around after two young children helped keep my weight at this level.

So, with my husband now back at work and life settling down, was it finally time to eat fresh wholesome food in moderation and exercise regularly?

Of course not!

Now was the time to join a university research study during which participants ate only 800 calories a day of 'delicious' meal-replacement shakes and bars. A friend of mine had done it and lost 10 kilos. She'd put it all back on, but I ignored that inconvenient fact. I submitted myself to the researchers' needles and tests and measurements and got started on their diet. I lasted two weeks and I lost the same 4 kilos I'd been losing and putting back on again for the previous few years.

And then my uncle's bowel cancer came back. He had fought it successfully for two years, but suddenly it was everywhere: back in his liver, but also in his lungs and his stomach. There would be no more treatment. My two sisters and I flew interstate to see him. He was pale and bloated and tired but still great company. We spent a wonderful day with him, laughing and telling stories – my family's favourite way to whittle away time. I told him I loved him and that he had been a great uncle, and then my sisters and I left to fly home, knowing we would never see him again.

When I got on the plane I couldn't get the seatbelt around my stomach.

Now was it time to fulfil that promise I'd made to myself in the hospital car park? Was it time to stop killing myself with food and be a good role model to my children?

Yes, actually, it was.

Chapter Three

118 kilos

Now it was time to call a nutritionist.

I was forty-seven years old. I'd spent thirty-four years struggling with my weight – thirty-four years of diet shakes and weight-loss books and slimming teas and thousand-dollar programs run by skinny twenty-year-olds with no training who had never had a weight problem in their thin, short lives. Yet I had avoided doing the sensible thing. I'd always gone for the solution that had the words *fast* or *quick* or *easy* (or preferably all three) in the title.

I'd always chased the miracle cure because, secretly, I thought there was something wrong with me and only a miracle would work. I thought about food all the time. All the time. When was I going to get it? How could I get it? Would anyone notice if I had a second helping? A third helping? Was that small tray of cheese the only food at the party? Would my husband find the stash of chocolate under the bed? Would the kids discover I'd eaten all their Easter eggs and replaced them with new ones, again?

I felt panic in situations where I couldn't control how much food I would get and when I would get it. And yet, with all my eating, the weird thing was that I was never satisfied. Never. No amount of food was actually ever enough. After finishing a big meal I would start thinking, almost immediately, about the next thing I could eat.

Of course this waxed and waned over the years. Sometimes, when I had been particularly happy, food hadn't been so dominant, such as when I was caught up in a writing project, or falling in love with Russell or on a big family holiday with the kids. But it had been waxing much more than waning in the past few years, with my cancer, then my stressful job, then my husband's cancer and breakdown.

And some of the so-called miracles had actually worked – for a bit. I had sometimes lost weight and even got down to a size 14 or even a 12, starving every step of the way. But I had always put it all back on again.

The only time I actually stopped thinking about food was after my own cancer, when I fell apart. I would wake up each morning with one thought in my head: *What terrible thing is going to happen today?* And I'd ask that one question over and over all day until I went to bed where I would lie awake asking it all night before slipping into a few hours of restless sleep full of dreams where horrible things happened to me and my family and I couldn't stop them. My cancer had come at the end of a very stressful period in our lives. My father had died, I'd been retrenched from my previous job and I'd been diagnosed with cancer all in the space of eighteen months. Prone to anxiety attacks since my twenties, I was now living with constant dread and terror.

I finally found relief with anti-anxiety medication, counselling and time – good, old-fashioned time. And as few bad situations don't have the sliver of good, the sliver I took from that experience was that it was actually possible for me to not focus on food every waking minute. I hoped a nutritionist would help me find that happy place again – but without the cancer diagnosis this time.

So, there I was. Done with gimmicks and contacting a nutritionist. Okay, emailing her. Email felt so much less immediate than phoning. I was hoping to put off the alfalfa sprouts as long as I could because I knew it was going to be tough. I knew I was about to lose all my crutches and comforts and coping mechanisms and I had nothing much to replace them with.

I started typing and told the nutritionist I wanted to learn how to eat normally and lose weight. I told her I was very committed. I didn't tell her I was also terrified.

But the biggest motivation of all wasn't me. It was our children. I'd watched my mother go on and off diets all her life and had seen how her confidence was totally connected to her weight. With my mother's encouragement, I had started dieting at the age of thirteen. I didn't want that for my kids. I wanted them to have a happy relationship with food and to not see it as an enemy that had to be constantly battled and defeated. That it was just, well, food.

I pressed send.

I hadn't chosen just any nutritionist – one I could dump when it got too hard, one with whom I could cancel appointments and then eventually say, 'I'm so busy. I'll call you to make the next appointment when things settle down,' and never call them again, like I'd done on so many other weight-loss programs. The skinny twenty-year-olds would leave messages about how much they missed me, messages that were easy to ignore. They didn't miss me. They missed my wallet.

Aprille, the nutritionist, would not be so easy to ignore.

I had chosen her for one big reason: we knew each other. Our kids went to the same primary school. We lived in the same neighbourhood, shopped at the same shops and had friends in common. Our families went to the same parks and markets and festivals; we sat on committees together and would see each other regularly at the school gate.

There would be no blowing Aprille off when it all got too hard.

The other reason I chose Aprille was because she wasn't a skinny twenty-year-old. Sure, she was skinny. Tiny. I could fit her into one leg of my pants. And she glowed with good health. Literally glowed, like there was a Roman candle inside her. But surprisingly, for someone who now ran marathons and went on epic 100-kilometre bike rides, she had been overweight when she was a teenager. When she was a new mum she had got her weight under control and then gone back to uni to study nutrition. She had just graduated and started a business teaching people like me how to manage their food.

And she was no pushover. Aprille has a smile that could light up a Christmas tree but she was also fiercely focused with a wicked sense of humour and a finely honed bullshit detector. She was the one for me.

She responded to my email and suggested that we set up a time to meet at *my* house. Why? I wondered. So she could look in my cupboard? But I reluctantly agreed. After all, this time I was serious. And besides – all the really bad food was under my bed.

When she rang the doorbell at seven o'clock on the Friday night of our first meeting I seriously thought about running out the back door. Just for a split second. But I didn't. I answered the door and welcomed her into my very messy house. I was embar-rassed by the mess. Another part of my life I was ashamed of. Another part of my life I couldn't get under control.

She got out her scales and, yep, I was still 118 kilos. Then she sat down at my kitchen table with me and my husband there to support me. The three of us talked for an hour about my history of dieting, my goals and her approach. She asked me, on a scale of one to ten, how committed I was to losing weight.

'Ten,' I told her without flinching. Not because I was looking forward to alfalfa sprouts, but because if this didn't work I was out of options.

I expected Aprille to lecture me about calories in and calories out. About how if I ate less and exercised more I would lose weight. I'd heard it all before, knew it didn't work, but I was still hoping she had some magic way to make it happen this time.

The first thing she said was to forget everything I had ever heard about losing weight. And then she didn't talk about calories, she talked about insulin. About how high-carb foods spike your insulin, which is a fat-storing hormone. She told me how cutting out high-carb foods completely would even out my blood sugar, reduce my cravings, that I would eat less and the weight would just fall off.

'Oh, like Atkins and the CSIRO diet,' I told her. 'I've done them both and they didn't work. I just ended up craving pasta until I was so hungry I'd eat it raw because I couldn't wait the ten minutes for it to boil.'

She shook her head. 'Atkins is low-carb, high-protein. This is low-carb, high-fat.'

I pictured myself eating a bucket of butter for breakfast.

Aprille qualified her high-fat statement. 'It's called high-fat but it isn't really. Fat isn't the main part of the diet. It's just a higher level of fat than you would normally eat; than the food pyramid with its six to eleven serves of grains per day tells you to eat. The pyramid is wrong. Everything you have ever heard about losing weight is wrong.'

I took a moment to digest this. 'But doesn't fat make you . . . umm . . . you know . . . fat?'

Aprille smiled. 'That's a myth. Your body needs fat. And it's very sating. It makes you feel full. The obesity epidemic started when the low-fat craze began. Low-fat foods don't fill you up, and they're packed full of sugar to make them taste better. Everything you eat from now on will be full fat.'

'Seriously?'

'Seriously. Butter, full-fat milk, cheese and yoghurt. And nothing processed. Home cooking. I don't want you eating any-thing out of a packet. Can you manage that?'

I turned to Russell. Russell does most of the shopping and cooking in our household, and is a far better cook than I am. He nodded.

Aprille put my first week's menu on the table. 'No potatoes, rice or corn. They're very high in carbs. No wheat at all. Wheat is the only food that crosses the brain-barrier. It's very addictive and spikes cravings. In fact, you aren't to eat any grains at all. Or sugar. Lots of vegies, with eggs, fish and meat. And you're to have lots of good fats, like coconut oil and avocados. Drink water and take vitamin D.'

I looked at her menu. Breakfast was eggs or a homemade almond-meal banana muffin. Dinner was protein, vegies and good fats. Snacks were nuts or yoghurt. Lunch was *weird*: lunch was leftover dinner.

Aprille explained. 'Lunch is no longer bread or pasta based. Make an extra amount of dinner and have the leftovers the next day for lunch. Simple.'

Aprille said this was not a diet. It was a lifetime approach to good health and nutrition. It all looked very doable, and there wasn't an alfalfa sprout in sight.

She asked me about the exercise I was doing. Instead of looking sheepish and saying something vague about walking, as I usually did when asked that question by a health professional (yeah right – walking to the fridge and back), I was able to look her in the eye and say that I was working out at a gym twice a week and seeing a personal trainer once a week.

And it wasn't a lie. It was true.

Instead of having one fierce woman in my life, I now had two. I told Aprille about Mischa. Mischa was no twenty-something skinny personal trainer with perfect cheekbones in pink Lycra – though actually she was very trim and did have pretty damn good cheekbones and she did like pink. Mischa was an ex-champion boxer who ran her own boxing studio in the next suburb. I'd started taking my son there at the beginning of the year after he'd done some boxing in a fitness class and decided he wanted to do more. We were desperate to get him into a sport so agreed and found Mischa's gym on the internet.

I'd had an image of a boxing studio being full of tattooed ex-cons and street kids, without a brain cell to rub together between their cauliflower ears. I thought a gym run by a woman would be safer and nicer. I was wrong about boxing being for knuckleheads, but I was right about Mischa's gym. My son and I both loved it from the moment we stepped through the pink doorway. There were lots of tattoos but also lots of women and kids training, though some of the women had more tattoos than the men and were deadlier.

On our first visit we saw a woman in her thirties sparring in the ring. Her grunts echoed off the old warehouse roof and her punches were ferocious. She came and said hello after her session. That's the thing about Mischa's: everyone comes and says hello. The boxer's name was Diana Prazak. She told us what a great gym this was, that she had trained in boxing gyms all over the world and this was the best. My son loved his first class and we kept going back.

Pretty soon he was going twice a week. 'When I grow up I'm going to be a fighter,' he started telling me on the car ride home. *You already are, my darling*, I would answer silently, thinking about how he had coped when both Russ and I had cancer. We started going three times a week.

And I would sit there watching my son and everyone else work out, telling myself that I was now working full-time and studying and didn't have time to go to the gym. Seriously. I was at a gym three times a week. Right there. Not near it or driving past it or next door to it. Inside it, sitting on my backside, playing on my phone and watching my son. Finally a thought dawned on me. I'm at a gym! Three times a week!

Sheepishly I asked Mischa if she would mind if I started working out. She thought it was a great idea and so the next time I took my son I wore my size 26 track pants and sat on the exercise bike in the corner and pedalled for five minutes. And it nearly killed me. Then I put on some gloves and punched a bag for another five minutes. Then I lay down on a mat and tried to do a sit-up. Just one. One single, tiny sit-up. I strained and heaved and sweated like a pig. Nope. Not even one. I could lift my head off the mat and that was it. It wasn't a sit-up as much as a neck-up.

I was mortified. Was I that unfit? But none of the boxing guys and gals laughed at me, or even stared at me. And my son didn't mind either. He was proud of me for working out. And I was proud of him too; he was working so hard. One day, after one of my fairly short workouts, Diana came over for a chat and said that she had been watching my son and that he was getting good. I told him after his class and he grew six inches taller. Diana wasn't just mucking around in the ring to get fit or learn self-defence, she was the current WBC Super-Featherweight World Champion. There aren't many sports where a world champion would take the time to watch a beginner. But that's boxing. That's Mischa's.

My son and I went to see Diana fight, our first trip to a professional match. We were there with families, grandparents, kids. Diana dominated from the second round but her opponent had guts and skill and got a few good hits in. The ref called it off in the fifth round after a series of savage punches from Diana. Her opponent begged to keep going, the crowd booed the end of a good fight and Diana did her trademark leap through the air into the arms of her trainer. My son and I were both hooked. In other sports you try to hit a ball over a net or run faster than someone else. In boxing you try not to get punched in the face. It's as simple as that. The stakes are high and all you have is your training, your courage, your wits and your mental toughness. It's raw and it's addictive.

So, I kept wearing my size twenty-six track pants and sitting on that poor bike. The bike was against the far wall next to the ring, so every time I worked out I got a free show watching all the boxers spar. In the ring you can't hide your true personality. Your timidity, your desperation, your dive-in-and-swing-wildly style or your hang-back-and-wait approach to life all show. Some of the boxers at Mischa's spar with a look of terror or determination or defeat on their face; my son spars with a huge goofy grin from ear to ear. A film-maker came and made a short film at the gym, and my son was cast as a young boxer who was nasty and not very skilled. It was hard work for him to look bad at boxing; it was even harder for him to remember not to smile that goofy grin of his.

It wasn't long before I was doing thirty minutes of bike-riding without a break, enjoying my free boxing show and watching my son get better and better. My backside, which is square – seriously who has a square backside, I looked like a middle-aged version of SpongeBob SquarePants – was beginning to look smaller and rounder.

So, I took the big plunge. I started training one-on-one with Mischa once a week.

Mischa, the former champion boxer, was tougher than the stationary bike in the corner. She made me squat and lift weights and punch – so much punching. During the first training session the studio started to spin, and not in a good fun-park kind of way – more of an *I'm-going-to-throw-up* kind of way.

But I kept training. There have been times in my life when I have been very fit, and every so often working with Mischa I would feel a moment of muscle memory. It was fleeting, but it was there. When I was doing sit-ups (not neck-ups anymore, real fair-dinkum sit-ups) my core muscles would kick in and I would feel strong, stable and powerful. It would only last for a second but suddenly my body would remember the girl who had set a school record in javelin, been in the top netball team and had loved to run and run and run. Then the moment would pass and I would go back to heaving my sea of blubber around, but knowing those muscles were there waiting to be set free.

Now I had Aprille and Mischa in my corner, pardon the boxing pun. I had lost two whole kilos in the first week on Aprille's eating plan. I loved the fact that I didn't need to count calories or weigh my food. I also loved that it was based heavily on science. I found the website of one of the main proponents, a South African professor of exercise and sports science at the University of Cape Town called Tim Noakes. He used the term 'Banting' to describe this approach to eating. It comes from a pamphlet published in 1863 by English undertaker William Banting called

A Letter on Corpulence. The pamphlet outlined the Low Carb High Fat (LCHF) diet he followed to cure his obesity, and was in print until 2005. So, this wasn't even new science, it was old science that had got pushed aside by the low-fat processed-food approach to weight loss.

And Banting/LCHF was working. It was easier to walk up the steep platform to the station for my morning train, and my clothes started to feel looser. My exercise regime was going well too. Mischa had me running (well run-shuffling, but a kind of almost-running that would one day turn into running) and I was down to 111 kilograms according to Aprille's scales.

All I had to do was keep doing what I was doing. But I started to tell myself I couldn't do it. Would never do it. Was useless and hopeless and lazy. I started to sneak foods – sugary, wheatie foods like croissants and cupcakes. I missed the highs from eating sugar, and I really missed that heavy half-drugged feeling of filling up on bread and pasta. Eating Aprille's way was boring because it had no peaks and troughs. And going to the gym was hard. Before long I had started to put weight back on and had to regularly give myself a stern lecture. I would try really hard and lose weight the next week only to put it back on the week after.

Then I had an accident. An accident that wouldn't have happened if I'd been sticking 100 per cent to Aprille's eating plan. I was whipping some cream for a chocolate mousse. My chocolate mousse is a thousand times better than the Weight Watchers version – it's full of fresh eggs and whipped cream and melted dark chocolate. It wasn't anywhere on Aprille's meal plan but had snuck back into our Sunday family dinner. I was showing my son how to make it and was demonstrating how to put our electric hand-mixer together. What I forgot to show him was how to check the mixer wasn't plugged in and switched on before you insert the beaters. I stood for a moment watching the ring finger on my right hand whizz around inside one of the beaters before screaming and dropping the mixer on the kitchen floor. I looked down at my hand, and my ring finger was bent sideways. 'Go get Daddy,' I told my son as I grabbed my hand.

He ran out to the back garden and yelled, 'Daddy, come quick! Mummy's cut her finger off!' Russell rushed in looking paler than me. My finger wasn't cut off but it was dislocated, and I couldn't work for a few days or drive for a week. But I used it as an excuse to blow off the gym for a month. A month! And to eat anything I wanted. And all the weight I'd lost started to creep back on. And then my lovely husband got sick – not cancer-sick, just flu-sick, but he couldn't work for a week and I needed to step up and shop and cook as well as work and study and my finger hurt and I felt tired and old and fat and I JUST COULDN'T DO THIS.

So, I didn't. I stopped. I'd lost some weight. That was good, right? That was better than nothing. I'd improved my health a bit.

But I was so disappointed in myself. This time was supposed to be different; this time was supposed to work. This time I had been really serious, hadn't I? What was wrong with me? What was it going to take to get me to lose weight for good?

Aprille said, 'Just keep going. You don't have to be perfect all of the time – just eat well most of the time. It's about change over time not one big change. Be stronger than your excuses.'

Mischa said, 'Train when you're tired. Train when you're injured. Train when you can't be bothered, then when you get in the ring to fight and you're tired, injured and can't be bothered you can still fight.'

I didn't want to fight. I wanted to eat whatever I liked all day and to lie on the couch watching *Miss Fisher's Murder Mysteries* in the evening rather than going to the gym. I wanted my salted caramel cupcake and I wanted to eat it too. All of it. I began to resign myself to feeling fat and useless and stupid and lazy and hopeless for the rest of my possibly short life.

But then it happened. THE BIG EPIPHANY. It didn't come this time in a car park, or on top of a mountain or on a psychiatrist's couch.

I was lying in bed trying to sleep and thinking about why I couldn't stop eating. Willing THE SECRET to come. Because surely there was a secret to losing weight that I didn't know and everyone who had lost weight did know. 'What is THE SECRET?' I lay there chanting to myself.

'Why do I quit every diet?' I asked the ceiling and the lamp and the pile of messy clothes on my bedroom floor. 'Why do I quit? Why do I quit? Why do I quit?'

And then it came to me, as clear as the nose on my face.

I quit. When it got tough, as it always did, I quit. I could have given Weight Watchers Lady a second chance. I could have used all those gym memberships I had bought over the years. I could have stuck to one of the less whacky diets I had gone on.

But I didn't. I quit.

And now I was quitting Aprille and Mischa.

That was the BIG SECRET. That was THE EPIPHANY. When diets got boring and tough and when exercise got difficult and I was tired and stressed, I quit and I didn't go back. I'd play the soundtrack in my head that went, *I'm hopeless and lazy and fat and will never change*, and I'd take my bat and my ball and my chocolate mousse and I'd go home to watch TV and feel sorry for myself.

Along with THE SECRET and THE EPIPHANY came THE RESOLVE.

I was not going to quit this time. The towel throwing would stop right there and then.

I might fail and fail and fail again, but I would keep going. There would be lots of times when I would feel hopeless and think that I couldn't do it, but I would persevere. I would be a good role model for my children. I would stop endangering my health.

That is how I would succeed. Successful weight loss was not about committing myself to being healthy; it was about re-committing myself over and over and over again.

It was that simple.

I rolled over and fell asleep and had the best night's sleep I'd had in ages.

Chapter Four

111 kilos

The first thing I did the next day was buy a new set of bathroom scales. I needed to know what I weighed. Not constantly – with clothes, without clothes, before breakfast, after breakfast, before a bowel motion – the new scales weren't about obsessing about that little flashing number and calling myself good if the number went down or bad if it went up as I'd done on every other diet. But I needed to start weighing myself in between seeing Aprille every fortnight. Fourteen days was too long to go without knowing whether what I was doing was working.

The next thing I did was buy a new pair of runners. My runners were at least five years old and both my big toes were poking out of holes in the ends of them. Mischa had mentioned my sneakers in that way she has of not saying anything but just asking a question then raising an eyebrow. 'Are they your shoes for training?' Cue eyebrow lift.

I went to one of those shops where they measure your feet and get you to walk on a special sensor and then fit you properly. The young, thin attendant asked me what kind of exercise I would need the shoes for. 'Running,' I muttered, not having the guts to say boxing. Not that Mischa would call what I was doing boxing – punching at pads isn't boxing, not even close.

The attendant brought out a pair of fluorescent orange and pink sneakers and I fell in love with them. They were so bright and funky; if ever I went running on a dark night, got lost in a fog and fell down a cliff the police helicopter would easily be able to spot me. And they would fit in with all the pink at Mischa's. Then the attendant showed me the $200 price tag, which was allegedly their discounted price. When had runners got so expensive? The hole-poking sneakers had cost $80 and I'd thought that was expensive all those years ago. I handed over my credit card.

But there was one more thing I needed. Mischa had told me about a big-chested girl she trained who wore two bras and a tight T-shirt so she could skip. Boxers do a lot of skipping. Then Mischa had raised an eyebrow and looked at my very abundant chest.

I've always had big breasts. When I started university I'd lost a lot of weight because I was happy and doing theatre and meeting fun people and finally out of the hellhole that was the private girls' school my parents had paid a fortune for me to be miserable at. At that time in my life I was a size Double D. I told myself that D was for delicious, delightful, delectable. I loved my breasts back then. I wore a red bra under my 1950s op shop dresses and I remember one of my first partners, a gorgeous Italian boy, lying next to me after we had made love and saying, 'My God, you're beautiful.' He was looking at my breasts at the time.

But later, in my twenties, I started to put on weight again. Some women put weight on around their waists, or on their thighs or on their backside. Every chocolate bar I ate went straight to my breasts. My lovely Double Ds crept up to an E size. I told myself E was for excellent. E was for exceptional. E was for a little bit too big to be comfortable but still lovely.

Then in my early thirties E became F. F did not stand for fantastic. It stood for too big to run, too big to wear nice clothes and under-boob sweat. Lots and lots of under-boob sweat. Then I had my first child. Chuck in pregnancy hormones and lots more chocolate and my F cups became G cups. Yes, they do actually make G cups. They come from America and they cost a fortune. But I wasn't done there. Oh no. At thirty-nine I got pregnant again and knew straightaway I'd conceived when in one week my breasts went from a G cup to an H cup. I was so happy to be pregnant. Except for the H cup.

After giving birth my breasts didn't go down like most women's do. They stayed an H. To me, H stood for heavy and highly embarrassing. And they weren't even any good for breast-feeding; I was hopeless at it.

I went to see a surgeon about getting a breast reduction. He kept me waiting two and a half hours, gave a cursory apology for his lateness then told me he wouldn't touch me until my Body Mass Index (BMI) was down to 32. BMI is an indication of your body fat. It's calculated by your weight (in kilograms) divided by your height squared (in centimetres), and at 171 centimetres tall and 122 kilograms I had a BMI of 41.7. The ideal BMI range for adult women is 18.5 to 24.9. So, according to the surgeon, I would have to get my weight down to 93 kilos to have a BMI of 32 before he would operate. That or grow another 27 centimetres taller.

The reason I would have to wait, the surgeon said, was that breasts were like a football field. (Yes, he really said this.) And that, like a football field, they had an irrigation system of blood vessels to 'water' them. And my breasts were a very big football field and had therefore developed a very big watering system, so the chances of my having bleeding problems after the surgery were greatly increased. He also said he didn't want to operate at my current weight because it would be his work on display and the breasts would look much better if I was thinner. Did he think that after the surgery I was going to walk around naked with my new smaller-but-not-very-good breasts on display for all the world to see? Perhaps wearing a placard that said, *These not-very-good-but-smaller breasts are brought to you courtesy of an astoundingly arrogant surgeon from a highly expensive suburb in Melbourne?*

I didn't want to walk around naked; all I wanted to do was to wear bathers and buy normal clothes and not have back and neck pain all the time. I googled a lot of other surgeons and they were all the same. Not arseholes, I mean, but they all required prospective breast-reduction patients to have a BMI of 30–32. So, I was stuck with my gigantosaurus breasts for now. Another reason to lose weight so I could one day have the surgery. Though probably not with Football-Field Surgeon. I would find one who had a modicum of compassion and human decency.

If I was going to train seriously I needed to get a new bra, because my breasts were holding me back. But I kept putting it off. I hated bra shopping. I hated walking past the lacy slinky bras in the front of the shop to the fat-lady section at the back with the ugly thick-strapped bras that only come in beige. I hated being stuffed into bras that didn't fit, with the attendant shaking her head saying, 'I was sure that one would do it.' And I really hated having to look at myself in their floor-to-ceiling mirrors. Then, when I was far away from home on a writing retreat, I found myself walking past a bra shop and went in. No more excuses. I had the scales, I had the new sneakers. It was time for a new bra.

The Russian bra-shop owner shrieked and came running over when she saw me. 'Your girls are supposed to be up here,' she declared to everyone in the shop in a very loud voice, 'not sitting on your stomach!' Then she grabbed my bra straps and hoisted my breasts up so high I almost fell over backwards.

'We will get them up here!' she declared, like I was her greatest challenge.

She stood back and sized me up, then ushered me into a changing room and came back with one bra. Not seven like they do in most underwear shops, hoping that maybe one of them would be able to contain my massiveness. Russian Lady had one. And oh boy what a bra. It looked like it had come straight from a Soviet-era torture chamber. It was actually American (of course), and hugely expensive, but gosh did it get my girls to stand up and pay attention. It worked so well because it was made from extra-thick material and was very heavily stitched, but also because, I suspected, there had been a substantial amount of concrete poured into its seams during production. There would be no more jiggling at the gym. There would be no more saggy breasts resting on my huge stomach. There would be no more sagging full stop. Now I could skip. Now I could run without being a danger to myself or anyone in a one-metre radius. With my new shoes and wearing the concrete bunker, I was ready to train. Really train.

My son's boxing class went for an hour and a half. He had moved up from the kids' class and was now working out with adults. His trainer was quite young and was no gruff, yelling trainer. 'No, no, do it again,' he would say softly to my son and the others in his class. And they would. Over and over again. Footwork drill, set punches, scissor kicks with their feet in the air and their heads off the mat and the sweat pouring down their faces.

Ninety minutes was a long time for me to train. Usually I would do about thirty minutes then would goof off, play on my phone and watch my son. No more. If my son could train for an hour and a half three evenings a week, then so could I. The old warehouse where Mischa has her gym is down by the river. There's a path along the river from Mischa's to a big golden Buddhist statue that stands looking out across the water and the city beyond. It's 3 kilometres there and 3 kilometres back. Could I ever run all the way to that statue and back? After all, it was daylight savings and therefore sunny until quite late. When I was really fit during one of my boot-camp frenzies I could run 5 kilometres in thirty minutes. So, if I got that fit again it would take me about forty minutes to run 6 kilometres. Then there would still be time for some bike work, rowing, sit-ups and stretches to cool down.

Really? I was going to run to the statue and back? That was three bridges over the river away. I couldn't run. I shuffled. Maybe I needed to set a smaller goal, like the letterbox at the end of our driveway. But I knew I had all summer before it got too dark in the evenings. I had spunky new shoes and it was time to rock them. Okay, shuffle them.

So, I took my son to his class, told Mischa I was going for a run, ignored her raised eyebrow and set off. I ran out of Mischa's and through the alleyways that led down to the river. I had to pass three seafood wholesalers to get to the waterfront and boy do they smell at the end of a summer's day. I made it to the water and stopped to catch my breath and to get the scent of rotting fish out of my nostrils. Then I shuffled to the nearest tree and stopped to catch my breath. Then I did a bit more shuffling, going faster when a jogger or someone on a bike passed me and then slowing down when it was all clear.

I got to the first bridge and stopped again to catch my breath. Then I turned around and shuffled all the way back to the gym, stopping about fifteen more times on the way.

I was bright red and I didn't do too many sit-ups when I got back.

'Did you get to the statue, Mum?' my son asked.

'Not quite.'

'How far did you get?'

'The bridge.'

'Which bridge?'

'The first one.'

'Good job.'

'Thanks, honey.'

I stuck at it. I was determined to get to the statue. Each time I shuffled a little further and a little faster. The rest stops decreased and the length of time shuffling increased. My ankles hurt, my knees hurt, everything hurt. But soon I was making it to the second bridge. Then the third bridge. Then I made it to that giant golden statue. It was standing in a pool of stinking, fetid water, but damn it I was there. I had made it. I had ticked that box. Achieved that goal. Now all I had to do was keep sticking to the diet and keep running and I would be well on my way.

Chapter Five

102 kilos

Wouldn't it be a lovely fairy tale if I'd stuck to the diet and kept going to the gym? Smooth sailing from fat to thin, from chaos to control.

But changing the habits of a lifetime is rarely smooth. Or easy.

I know, I know, I know. I said I was serious this time. I'm sounding like a broken record, but I got tired, and my son fell off his scooter and hurt his shoulder and didn't go to boxing for a month, so I didn't go either, and the summer ended and it got dark in the evenings and I *really* like food. Have I mentioned that last part?

And to top things off someone put Super Glue on my scales, and on Aprille's scales, and on the scales at the gym. All three got stuck at 102 kilos and they wouldn't budge. And no matter how many times I threatened to smash my scales with a hammer it just stared back up at me with 102 in big red smiling numbers.

This was not fair. I was working hard and had lost 20 kilos. Twenty whole kilos. Have you tried lifting 20 kilos? It's heavy!

But no one had really noticed that I had lost weight. People would look at me and say, 'You're looking good.' Which translates as, 'You're still huge but not as enormously huge as you used to be.' My clothes did feel looser but not by a gigantic amount. And I was still battling cravings.

I wasn't exercising much, but I was sticking to my diet, which is actually 80 per cent of weight loss. I hadn't eaten any wheat for five months, and I hadn't touched sugar for two months. Not a grain. I was skipping breakfast and fasting till lunchtime every day as Aprille had suggested as a way to speed up the weight loss. I wouldn't have recognised a piece of pasta, a grain of rice, a cob of corn or a baked potato if they had chased me down the street, thrown me against a wall and held me at gunpoint.

But was I sticking to my diet? I mean really sticking to it? I wasn't snacking on cupcakes anymore, as I had been at the beginning of the diet, but my meals were still too big. This low-carb/high-fat diet isn't about measuring food or counting calories – which is great – but Aprille had set guidelines around the amount of food I could consume and I was eating far more than I was supposed to and sneaking nuts and cheese.

And I was still struggling with my night-time eating. I'm an insomniac and food in bed at night was a habit I had got into because I find it hard to sleep on an empty stomach. I wasn't going to bed with a packet of chocolate biscuits as I'd done when my husband was sick, but there was a bit of a nut and cheese festival going on in casa del bed that needed to stop.

Aprille even had me text her every morning for a week to let her know whether I had stuck to her no-food-after-8pm rule. I kept at it for a week, as promised, texting her my success every morning, then when the week was up I went straight back to enjoying my 10pm mini-meal.

Hence the Super-Glued scales. I think Aprille began to think I was deranged or deluded or not quite right in the head somehow. I kept saying I wanted to change and lose more weight, but my actions didn't change. I just kept bouncing between 102 and 103 kilos.

I like to look for inspiration on the internet, to read about other people who have successfully shed a lot of weight, perhaps in the hope that their willpower will electronically be instilled in me through the magic of the World Wide Web. One night, while enjoying my 'binner', which is what I had come to call this meal between dinner and breakfast, I read a blog by someone who had lost a lot of weight, and what she said really resonated. Unlike me, she had been a smoker and had given up the cigarettes by compensating with food. Instead of smoking in the evening she had sat on her couch watching TV and eating two Magnum ice-creams each night. She said that it had taken her three months of sticking to a Magnum-free diet to realise she would be okay without those two ice-creams.

Bam. World Wide Web magic. I realised I was still frightened of being without food. Eight months into this work with Aprille, 20 kilos down, and fear was still holding me back. I felt panicked if I couldn't be sure of when and where and how I was going to eat. Food had always equalled comfort and energy, and food calmed my anxiety. And none of those fears or needs had changed.

I wasn't always tired, stressed, anxious and frightened of being disconnected from food. So, what had happened to me? And I wasn't always overweight. For the first thirteen years of my life I was fit and active and food was just food. It didn't rule my every waking thought.

There was only one time, when I was a child, that I remember having a voracious appetite. It was when my family and I were living in Singapore. My dad had been transferred there by the bank he worked for. We went from the bland suburbs of Melbourne to living in an apartment on the twenty-first floor with views across the Java Sea. I went from a local government school, where boys and girls weren't allowed to play together because the school said the boys were too rough, to an international school with fifty-two different nationalities. It was all swimming pools and open-air food markets and lots of other expat kids from all over the world.

But when we were about a year into our three-year transfer I suddenly couldn't stop eating. I would sneak into the kitchen behind our amah's back and pour a packet of icing sugar into a bowl, add cocoa powder and butter, mix it together, and then eat the whole bowl of chocolate icing and still not feel full. Then one night as I was falling asleep I felt something wriggling at the back of my throat. I reached into my mouth and pulled out a tapeworm. My mother took me to the doctor the next morning and he made me swallow the biggest pill I have ever seen. Huge appetite sorted!

Oh, if only appetite control could be that easy again. If there was just one big pill I could take to be normal again.

When we came back to Melbourne I was thirteen and hitting puberty in a big way, I had lost touch with all my old friends and was going to yet another new school – my fifth. I was so sick of being the new kid. And I hated my new high school. A private girls' school that put the bore in boring. I missed Singapore so much I ached. Our apartment building had a huge swimming pool and I'd swum every afternoon after school for hours, had run every evening with my sister Ruth, and was on the netball team and in the athletics squad. I could do the 100 metres in fifteen seconds.

We arrived home in summer, but it was not the kind of summer I was used to. No hanging out with the other kids in the pool, playing in the deserted mansion next door, snacking on paw paw and rambutans, staying up till 3am every night of the school holidays roaming the streets or playing cards by the pool with friends from the building, and none of our expat parents even noticing that we weren't home because they were out at cocktail parties and were too drunk to care. In Australia it felt like there was just heat and lots of it, burning the grass in the empty backyard where I had no one to play with.

My new school sat atop a hill, looking down on everyone. The uniform was a blue blazer, blue dress and matching blue underpants – the latter presumably in case an ambulance driver saw them after we'd been hit by a bus and was distressed that they didn't match our uniform.

And not just any blue. Navy blue. One of the teachers once came tearing across the quadrangle screaming my name. What on earth had I done to cause such fury? She stopped in front of me panting and flapping her arms. 'Sarah Vincent. The ribbon in your hair is royal blue not navy blue. Take it out at once!'

That first year at my new school I went home each night and stuffed my pain down with chocolate biscuits and hours of TV cartoons, the result being that for the first time in my life I was overweight, and I didn't know what to do about it. I managed to make a friend at school but I think she was as depressed and lonely as I was. The only thing we really had in common was how much we both hated the school. One day when I was at her house she asked if she could borrow one of my school skirts to wear to a school music event. 'Of course!' I said, but when she tried it on it was far too big for her, which sent her and her mother into fits of giggles. That was the end of our friendship. Being hopeless at confrontation, I never told her how much she had hurt my feelings or gave her an opportunity to explain or understand how sensitive

I was about my weight. I just drifted away from her and then drifted through the next four years without a close friend or ally, yet again.

Food was a friend. But it was a fickle friend. I hated myself – overweight, lonely, boyfriend-less, never fitting in. Being a teenage girl, I focused a lot on my weight. Surely that was the root of all my problems? Surely if I lost weight I would be happy, get close friends, get a boyfriend, get better marks? Following my mother's example, I discovered dieting and went on the lose-five-pounds-in-five-days diet. You ate to a strict five-day schedule. One day was a scoop of vanilla ice-cream and a banana. Another day was an apple and a slice of plain toast. I can't remember the other three days. I did drop weight, but it all came back and brought friends with it. Not real live nice friends. Blubbery, cellulite, kilo friends.

My grades began to slip badly. I was failing all my subjects except English, and was shatteringly lonely. And I had no one to turn to for advice or comfort because we never talked about our problems in my family, probably because we had so many of them. My mother was bi-polar but was not on proper medication because she had yet to be diagnosed with it, and had quickly become addicted to taking sleeping pills and tranquillisers to try to control her mood swings. Dad meanwhile had a long-time drinking problem. Mum did get help much later in life and Dad did get his drinking more under control and became a terrific father and grandfather, but that was years away from this silent, lonely mess of a house.

It was even more silent than usual because my two sisters had left home by this stage and I had no buffer for my parents' misery. Mum was having another breakdown, and my dad's drinking was off the scale. I couldn't concentrate at school and was falling even further behind. Luckily for me I was still studying in an era when Year 12 consisted of an end-of-year three-hour exam for each subject. I managed to pull myself together and crammed a whole year's work into three weeks of intense revision before the exams. I have never worked so hard in my life. Driven by fear of failure and sensing that getting to university would be my only escape from the black shroud I had been wearing since Singapore, I drank a lot of coffee and divided my days into four-hour blocks of Chemistry, Maths and European History. I loved English and my English teacher too, so I didn't need to slot in too many hours on that subject. Somehow I fluked a C in European History and in Chemistry, and an A in Maths and English. I will never forget the look of shock on my chemistry teacher's face when I told her about my 68 per cent pass.

Finally I was free and vowed never to wear navy blue ever again. I was eighteen and headed off to Monash University to get an Arts Degree. I wanted to be a writer. I wanted to create people who were brave (unlike me), had friends (unlike me) and were the champions of their own lives (totally unlike me). But my desire to write wasn't just because I longed to say clever things on the page to compensate for the fact that in real life I was tongue-tied and shy. I loved words. I loved smashing them together or letting them slip and slide over each other. I loved beautiful words like *lilt*. I loved hard words like *kerb*. I loved ugly words like *mackerel* and silly words like *mushroom*. I loved hooking them together like carriages on a train and sending them down the track to see how fast they could go or how high they could climb.

But mostly I loved being in control and having things make sense, because in real life I had no idea what I was doing and had no control over anything.

Going to university was like someone turning on the lights again. All of a sudden there were interesting people and ideas and politics and music. I discovered student theatre. I got involved in the comedy revues at Monash. Especially the writing side. The sketches I wrote weren't brilliant but it was great fun. There were long rehearsals, all-night parties and friends. Real friends. I remember the first time someone hugged me when I was feeling down. I didn't know what I was supposed to do, so I just stood there with my arms at my sides letting her. We didn't hug in my family. My older sisters and I weren't close. My parents were both too lost in their addictions to notice our pain or help any of us or even just wrap their arms around us and ask if we were okay, which we weren't. But friendship isn't something you can get good at overnight. Always being the new kid, I was still keeping most people at arm's length and being too clingy and needy with the few I let get close. I wasn't good at boundaries. And I was too worried that I would lose these precious new friends, so I never said anything if they hurt my feelings. I couldn't get the balance right.

I also had no judgement when it came to choosing friends. I frequently mistook charisma for character. I was drawn to the life of the party, regardless of whether that person had a kind heart. Although I had some brilliant friends – kind, loving, smart, funny – I kept overlooking them for the flashy, showy, confident people I so longed to be like. And I had a terrible habit of completely dropping friends when my life moved on to another area. This is a habit I have only just broken now in my forties. Perhaps it was a survival tactic from going to so many schools or being an expat: it was easier to dump friends than to try to hang on to them. I didn't do it consciously, crossing people out of my address book as soon as I finished a show, moved house, started a new job or changed to a different course of study; I just moved on and stopped contacting them, happy playing with my shiny new friends who hadn't figured out what a neurotic mess I was yet.

It never occurred to me that my old friends would be hurt. I just assumed everyone did the same thing.

In my second year at Monash I moved out of home into an old Victorian house in Carlton for the princely sum of $40 a week in rent. I was happy for the first time in ages. And I was thin. I remember once being at uni all day and coming home late after a play rehearsal and realising I hadn't actually eaten anything at all including breakfast. I'd been too busy. I eventually dropped out of my Arts degree, got a job making beds at a hospital nearby and spent all my spare time doing student theatre. Luckily no one noticed that I wasn't actually a student anymore.

All was going well until I got a boyfriend. There were some lovely, sweet, gentle boys in the student shows I was doing, but my first boyfriend wasn't one of those, and our year together was a misery. Somehow I had got it into my head that love was supposed to be miserable. And along with all the misery he loved to comment on my weight. I'd started putting it back on again, just a few pounds, and not a day would go by without some snide remark from him about how he didn't go out with fat chicks.

Well, actually it turns out he did – the high-school student he was also dating was quite plump, but I didn't find out about her until just before Christmas. He was working as a Santa at a big department store and I had quit my bed-making job and got a job as his elf – better pay than making beds. I found a card from her celebrating their four-month anniversary. Needless to say Santa's grotto wasn't a happy place that particular Christmas. My solution was to eat. I still wasn't really any good at friendships. I didn't know how to ask for help from my friends. I just bottled things up.

But even if my friendships and my love life weren't progressing, my writing was. I applied for a scriptwriting course at the Victorian College of the Arts in Melbourne. It was based in the drama school and only accepted two people every year, so I was over the moon when I was selected. I began the course full of hope that a glittering career as a playwright awaited me.

I was wrong.

In the first year of the course I started suffering from panic attacks. Bad ones. As I mentioned, in my family we didn't ever deal with problems. We drank or took pills and muddled through. When we were just back from Singapore and I was having trouble sleeping my mother gave me my own bottle of the tranquilliser Serepax to help me sleep so that she didn't have to dish them out to me anymore. I felt so grown up.

When I started having panic attacks Mum took me to her GP, who prescribed more Serepax, plus a benzodiazepine sedative, Stelazine (a dangerous anti-psychotic medication used for anxiety) and an MAO inhibitor anti-depressant called Parnate.

'I have lots of patients on this combination,' the silver-haired GP told me happily. I took them because he seemed to know what he was doing, even though he was the GP who had got my mother hooked on Valium, which started her prescription-drug addiction when my sisters and I were little.

All three medications were addictive. I waded through the three-year course doped to the eyeballs. The drugs didn't make the panic attacks go away but I was hooked and couldn't stop taking them. There were times the attacks were so bad I couldn't leave the house. I couldn't work and only barely survived on my government study allowance. Still living in share houses, I would hide in my room most of the time and drag myself into school for my classes, shaking with fear and dreading an attack.

When I finally started counselling at the end of the first year of my course, they couldn't believe the cocktail of drugs I had been put on. It was like swatting a fly with a sledgehammer, they said.

A very old sledgehammer. MAO inhibitors were ancient when my GP prescribed them and they weren't any good for panic, plus there were much better drugs for anxiety that had been around for quite a while. But worse than being a useless ancient drug, Parnate was also dangerous. The GP had warned me that if I ate any foods that contained high levels of Tyramine, an amino acid that helps regulate blood pressure, I could have a sudden and dangerous increase in blood pressure that could be fatal. And what foods contain high levels of Tyramine? Cured meats such as salami, fermented cabbage such as sauerkraut, soy sauce, Vegemite (that one hurt, I love Vegemite) and broad beans. All of that I could live without but the last food on the list was difficult. Very difficult. It was my favourite food – cheese. Hard cheeses like cheddar and soft cheeses like blue cheese or camembert – my favourites – were an absolute no-no. As was alcohol.

One of the other drugs he had me on, Stelazine, is a nasty drug that can cause permanent movement disorders and death. It can't be mixed with alcohol. I wasn't a big drinker, so giving up was easy, but it wasn't great for my anxiety to know I was taking two drugs that could kill me.

My counsellor helped me get off the drugs but it took three years. I went three years without cheese! That's how scared I was of the drugs. She also tried to help treat my anxiety by unearthing the reasons I was so frightened, which did little to help me. We would trawl through my childhood and tease apart the reasons I was afraid to sit in a theatre or go to parties and why I hated being in crowds. Was I afraid of success? Why did I have problems with my mother? (Erm, because she got me hooked on tranquillisers at thirteen for a start.) Sometimes the counsellor and I would sit in silence for an hour while I listened to her clock tick and couldn't think of anything to say.

I now know that anxiety is just plain fear. It is the fight-or-flight response gone haywire. For me, being in the moment, pushing myself to sit with the fear and still do all the things I want to do and seeing the fear as just thoughts in my head that can't hurt me is the way to manage it. Anxiety is just the negative catastrophising 'what ifs' that your mind throws up among the many thousands of thoughts it spews out every day. For some reason an anxious mind gets stuck on those negative 'what ifs' and plays them over and over like a broken groove in a record. History and family and personality do play a part, but only to help you understand how you became anxious. I believe that the key out of anxiety, or to making it manageable, is not psychoanalysis but a counsellor who specialises in anxiety, being in the moment and letting those negative thoughts be and not engaging with them. It took me years and several counsellors and much better drugs to find this all out.

But of course this is with the perspective of almost fifty years of living. Then I was twenty-two and terrified and on scary drugs. My life was very small and very tentative. I graduated from the course but I couldn't go to my graduation ceremony because of my panic attacks. I got a part-time job in the laundry of a nursing home because that was all I could manage, and I wrote and wrote and wrote. In between washing urine-soaked sheets I had a lot of plays performed at La Mama Theatre and other small venues around Melbourne. Despite my constant panic I was slowly building a bit of a name for myself, but when you can't sit in a theatre because you are terrified of having an attack, it makes constructing a serious career in the theatre really hard. Sometimes I wouldn't have a panic attack for weeks or even months. Then they would come back and my life would shrink back to my writing, my flat and those thousands of yellowing sheets.

I had some friends, but none I was really close to. I was still not good at asking for help or sharing my problems and, to be really honest, at being there for friends when they needed help, so life was again pretty lonely. And I had sworn off men, finally realising that I'd always gone for the bad boy at a party, and that until I could be trusted to go for someone decent I should just steer clear of men altogether.

I was now at the casino working as a valet captain parking the cars of problem gamblers and *Underbelly* drug barons, and going on random crash diets. I remember eating tomato and avocado for a whole month. I can't remember why; I probably read about it in a magazine. There was also a packaged-food diet, which involved driving to a suburb miles away and picking up a bag of food for the week, which cost hundreds of dollars I couldn't afford.

I changed part-time jobs again, this time to doing data entry at a university alumni office. I moved to the western suburbs of Melbourne to a tiny house with no heating and an outside bathroom right on the train line (the house, not the bathroom – that would have been embarrassing). Have you ever had a shower in winter in a small wooden room tacked onto the back of a small freezing house? I've never been so cold and I never got used to the mile-long 3am freight train that lumbered past each night making every window in the house shake. But my playwriting was still going well. I had two professional productions and two commissions. I moved house again, to one with an inside bathroom and heating (oh, the luxury) and I changed jobs. I got part-time work at a local library as a customer service officer – surprisingly, an associate diploma in scriptwriting from the Victorian College of the Arts doesn't lead to a stable employment future.

One night a group of three forty-year-old librarians I was working with, who had heard I was having singing lessons, invited me to a musical get-together near my house. I almost didn't go. I was a thirty-three-year-old playwright whose plays had been performed all around Australia. What was I doing hanging out with a bunch of cardigan-wearing middle-aged librarians?

I decided in the end that I'd go, but I promised myself that if anyone brought out a recorder or got the slightest bit nude I was out of there. As soon as I arrived a recorder was actually produced, but not an ordinary recorder. Trevor was an expert in playing medieval instruments and had an amazing collection. We listened to him play some mellow haunting music and he told us about the concerts he had coming up with his orchestra that specialised in old instruments. A very nice cake was served by the host, Barry, whose two young children were dancing around to Trevor's music and I was beginning to think I had misjudged these three middle-aged librarians, when Barry suggested that Russell play one of his own songs. Russell, who was forty and had receding hair, picked up his Maton guitar. I braced myself. I thought we were going to be doing covers not listening to a balding man sing about love and life and walking along the sand under the moon longing for his lost love who had left him sad and lonely. I looked at the clock. When would this be over?

Russell started playing and singing. The song was called 'Love Letters from Alma Road'. It was about a man whose wife had left him and then started sending him love letters. It was beautiful. As he sang a door opened in my sorry, sad, broken little heart and I felt light flow from him into me. I'm not talking a metaphoric imaginary beam of light. I mean a full-on, real shaft of powerful white light coming from him into my heart. I didn't see it so much as feel it. It was so powerful it almost knocked me off my chair. I walked home in a daze and told my flatmate I had just fallen in love with a forty-year-old librarian.

I decided to take it slow and not rush into anything, because I didn't even know his last name, and there was my arsehole romance radar to consider. He might be a great songwriter but he was probably a creepy loser. So, as we worked together I watched him and chatted with him and got to know him. After months of research I concluded: 1. He was handsome. 2. He was funny. 3. He was very kind. 4. He never bitched or gossiped. 5. Everyone liked and respected him. And 6. He was single.

Single? Really? Why weren't there women lining up around the block for this guy? Talking to Russell became the highlight of my week. I knew exactly which shifts he worked and when we would coincide. I always made sure I looked my best on those days.

One night I went to a house-warming party a co-worker at the library was having, hoping he would be there too. I spotted him chatting to Kim, a colleague, and squeezed through the crowds of people to join them. When Kim drifted off Russell and I stayed together, chatting about music and theatre and TV shows we liked. I couldn't help noticing that with his shaved head he looked more than a little like the uber-cool Paul Kelly, and that he had a lovely smile. Just then he lifted a curl that had fallen across my face and tucked it behind my ear. Startled, I spent the next hour wondering if that meant he liked me or whether he just didn't like untidy hair.

Towards the end of the evening Kim rejoined us, along with a couple of other colleagues, and Russell suggested going out for a coffee. To my disappointment they all jumped at the chance and the four of us piled into his car. Russell drove us to a cafe in Carlton where we had cappuccinos, and then dutifully drove everyone home. I thought this would be my chance to make my move, but Kim, who clearly knew nothing about the white shaft of light or my now desperate love for Russell, managed to score the front seat and told Russell to drop me off second, which meant that there would be no chance to find out if the hair-tucking incident was due to mutual attraction.

Russell and I continued our friendly chats at work but there were no more coffees suggested. And then I was offered another job. Much better pay than the library and using my writing skills working in the fundraising office at the same university where I had done data entry. It was an offer too good to refuse and nothing seemed likely to ever happen with Russell, so I took the new job and left.

Months went by. Months and months of me dropping by the library occasionally when I knew he'd be there but lacking the courage to make a move. Until one night I had a dream. In it I was sitting in a theatre watching a play when suddenly a dear friend who had committed suicide a few months before appeared beside me. 'You're alive!' I said to him. My friend smiled at me and said simply, 'Life is short,' and disappeared. The dream then switched to Russell and me married and tucking our two children into bed. I woke up with a gasp.

I got up that morning, put on make-up and my best outfit, tried to make my insanely curly hair look respectable and went to work, knowing what I had to do. On the way home from the office I went straight to the library, where Russell was at the front counter busy serving a customer. I waited anxiously in the queue while he scanned the lady's books, then hopped from one foot to the other while he helped a man with some DVDs. Should I have grabbed a book? Was I being too obvious just queueing up empty-handed to talk to him? I looked around for something to borrow. There was a book on the table near me about renal-function disorders and another about the history of crop harvesting. Neither of them seemed helpful to the current situation. The DVD man left and I stepped up to the counter bookless.

Russell seemed genuinely delighted to see me and we chatted at the counter for ages. I kept standing aside so he could serve customers, wishing them away so I could go back to talking to him. I laughed, I joked, I flirted but, God help me, I lost my nerve. I just couldn't ask him out. I kept telling myself that I had nothing to lose but my dignity, but the response in my head was always, *Yes, but that's all you've got.* Russell walked away from the counter to do some work and, deflated, I turned to go.

Just as I was about to leave he came back and handed me a piece of paper. It had his phone number on it.

We're married now with two kids. Sometimes dreams do come true. *Thank you, my friend; I hope wherever you are you are at peace. You would have loved Russell.*

Russell was far from the bad boy I used to go for. Not only did he never make jibes about my weight, he loved me just as I was. And feeling all loved up and with a new job, I made the reckless decision to buy a house. It's something I am still so ashamed of – not the house, I mean, but how I came to own it.

I had just been to Greece and Turkey with a dear friend, and while we were there my credit card hadn't worked. Without hesitating she had maxed out her own credit card to lend me $1000 for food and accommodation. Instead of repaying her the moment we got back, I saw the house up for sale and bought it, then emailed her and said, 'Great news. I've bought a house! Won't be able to pay you back for ages.'

Nice one. I still shudder at the memory. Along with being a bad friend who wasn't there for my friends when they needed me, and a cold friend who dumped people whenever I had shiny new friends, I was also a spectacularly selfish friend at times. Friendship is still a work in progress for me. Amazingly she forgave me, which says a lot about her. I don't deserve a friend like that.

When I walked into the bank with an $8000 deposit, which today would make any manager fall off their chair laughing, I was quickly made the proud owner of a crumbling house in West Footscray. And apart from moments of terrible selfishness, life was good. I owned a house, I had a lovely boyfriend and I had a career doing business writing. And then the cherry on the top: I fell pregnant. I was elated. Having children is the best thing I have ever done, but in all honesty it's also one of the hardest. The fact is that if you ever want to put on a lot of weight, completely lose your self-esteem and look awful – have a baby. In fact, have two. Pregnancy and sleepless nights and working and being a mum equals a lot of kilos. Add some cancer to the mix and you've got lots and lots of kilos.

And I stopped doing creative writing. When I was about to go on my first maternity leave I remember thinking that I would have plenty of time to write. I didn't write at all for FIVE YEARS. The only thing that got me writing again was my cancer. Another sliver of good that came from that dark time.

When the doctor told me I had bowel cancer, three thoughts went through my head. The first was, *Thank God it's me and not the kids*, as if some cancer bullet had been aimed at my family and had hit me and not them. It doesn't make sense but being told you have bowel cancer at forty-one doesn't make sense either.

The second thought was that I must make things up with Russell's daughter from his first marriage. She was nine when I first came on the scene and had long given up on getting her parents back together, so she happily accepted me. She was desperate for brothers and sisters and would give me drawings of her holding hands with her imaginary siblings. Like Russell she was very funny, kind and caring, and we got on like a house on fire when she came to stay each week. But as time went on and her imaginary siblings became real siblings, things began to deteriorate. I was suddenly a tired and grumpy mother and she was suddenly a grumpy teenager who hated coming to our house. And I didn't have the energy or stamina to deal with the tension between us so I focused on my own child.

As she got older we drifted apart and she stopped coming over. She would call to speak to her father and they would catch up once a week, but I took myself out of the picture. She was miserable at school (which I didn't know) and I was just plain miserable and it felt as if we couldn't find a way through our separate misery to help each other. The truth is, though, that I missed her. And when I was diagnosed with cancer I began making an effort to see her. Instead of passing the phone straight to Russell when she called and asked to speak to him and only him, I would make her chat with me. I began inviting her over and she came happily. The distance between us quickly disappeared and pretty soon she was having dinner with us at least once a week and no one was happier than my two kids, who worshipped her and loved seeing more of her. She had grown into a beautiful, funny, confident young woman and I am so proud to say that we have become good friends again.

My third thought in that doctor's room was that I couldn't die yet because I hadn't published a book. Even though I hadn't written a word in five years I still longed to write. And not plays anymore. I wanted to go back to my original idea of writing novels. I saw that the deadline for applying to do a course at RMIT University in Professional Writing and Editing was looming and I quickly put together a submission portfolio and dropped it off on my way to hospital to have my surgery. It looked like a practical course, had great teachers and a huge list of published authors as graduates, but I wondered if they would be reluctant to accept a now forty-two-year-old working mother who would be much older than all the other students and would only be able to fit in one subject per semester. At that rate it would take me years to complete the course and I could be in my fifties when I was finished.

A month later I had an interview and then got a wonderful letter saying I had been accepted into the course. And when I turned up for my first class it was full of mature-age students like me. By the time I graduated – at forty-nine (not yet fifty, but close) – I was submitting stories and articles to journals and had started being published in anthologies and placing in writing competitions. I was writing every day and even had my new job working at the amazing Writers Victoria, a job I absolutely loved. I got to work with wonderful dedicated people, and to be with writers and talk to writers and be among writing every day.

One day in class my fiction teacher Dr Olga Lorenzo was talking about her many students who had been published and had won awards as an example to us of focusing on our careers. One of my fellow students asked Olga if she could ever tell which of her students would be successful in the future.

'Of course,' Olga said.

That same student, as quick as a flash, asked who in our class would be published. Olga waved her question aside and said, 'Oh come now, you'll all be successful.' But then she stopped and looked straight at me. 'Sarah will be published,' she said firmly.

Everyone looked at me and I felt myself go bright red. Olga said it again. 'Sarah will be published.'

I worked twice as hard after that. I had to prove Olga right.

My panic attacks were still present but the new medication I started after the cancer was amazing and helped keep them to a manageable dull roar. I even had friends. Not people I was stuck with, or felt judged by, or who were mean. And not friends I was too intense with, too needy and demanding or cold and aloof with. I had real, loving, close, balanced friendships. I had some amazing women in my life whom I treasured. And I hoped that I was now as good a friend to them as they were to me.

I was also better at fitting in. I got on well with everyone at work and had made some fantastic new friends there. I was getting closer to the other writers in my course, I was in a great writing group that came out of a short course on Young Adult writing I did through Writers Victoria, plus I was much less awkward and tongue-tied among the school mums and dads. And I had grown very close to my sisters – something that had happened slowly once we had all moved out of home and had forged our own lives. My two sisters were my rocks when Russell was sick. I couldn't have got through his sickness without them. And our kids were doing really well and we were seeing heaps of Russell's daughter.

With Russell and I both now well, the only thing left for me to do was to keep losing weight. But despite feeling happier than I'd ever felt before, the weight loss had come to a grinding halt. I decided to get tough with myself. Aprille and I went through all my eating and came up with a stricter plan. I was to text her my weight every morning to tell her how I had done the day before, focusing in particular on breaking the habit of my night-time eating. I stuck to it rigidly for three weeks and broke the 102 mark. I even got down to just under 100. And then I fell off the wagon. For three days I ate like a mad thing and put it all back on again. Corn chips and ice-cream and chocolate. When it was time to weigh myself I barely had the courage to look down at the number on the scales.

I was back to 102.

Chapter Six

102 kilos (still!)

I hated being fat. I thought about how fat I was every day. And then I thought about how much I hated it and how much I hated myself for being so fat. And I know you're not even supposed to use the word 'fat' – you're supposed to say 'overweight' or 'robust' or 'horizontally challenged' or something – but when you're the one who's overweight you get to call it like it is. 'Fat' is certainly a nicer word than the medical term 'morbidly obese'.

If you've ever wondered what it's like to be morbidly obese, let me fill you in.

First of all, it's embarrassing. When I'd run into someone I hadn't seen for ages, they didn't know where to look. They looked at the floor, their shoes, an interesting poster on the wall – anywhere but at the suit of blubber I was now wearing. Or worse, they just stared at me in disbelief.

Clothes didn't fit. Clothes made for my size had really long arms and really long legs. Do our arms and legs grow longer when we get fat? Do we turn into orangutans? Of course we don't. Clothes makers are just lazy. They take a 'normal' sized outfit and make it bigger all over and then slap a size XL label on it.

When shops do make clothes specially for fat ladies, apparently we love three-quarter-length sleeves, with little straps and buttons on them to keep them in place. We're also mad for three-quarter-length pants. Perhaps the designers think we want to make ourselves look smaller by wearing shorter clothes. Or perhaps they are just trying to save on material.

Along with three-quarter-length attire apparently we love purple swirly tops. And green swirly tops. And red swirly tops. We're mad for swirls. Do they think swirls will make us look thinner? Or that our heads are so messed up we need this reflected in our attire?

It's not just clothes that don't fit. When I hit 122 kilos I couldn't even get my washing-up gloves on; I had to go up to the large size. I had put on so much weight I now had fat hands. And fat feet. I went up to a size 9½ shoe. I used to be a 7½. Getting older and having kids makes your feet spread, but two sizes? I felt like a fat-handed big-footed freak, in swirly three-quarter-length pants and tops with little buttons holding up my sleeves.

But buying clothes wasn't the hardest part of being so huge. At my heaviest I had trouble getting out of chairs, especially out of soft furniture such as the sofa or off my bed. I would have to rock back and forth like an old person to get enough momentum to stand up. That's fine when you're home alone, but not so fine when you're in a room full of people.

Oh, but that wasn't the worst thing. I also couldn't bend down to tie my shoelaces. I had to sit on the bed and flip a foot up onto the mattress to attempt it. Or I had to get my kids or Russell to do them up. And I had to get pedicures because I couldn't reach down to cut my own toenails. The occasional pedicure is lovely but not when they are essential and cost $40 a pop.

But come to think of it, that also wasn't the worst thing. I hated the way I looked so much I did all I could to avoid mirrors. Whenever I caught sight of myself, in a shop window, or in a restaurant bathroom that had a floor-to-ceiling mirror, or the most horrible place of all – in a change room with stark fluorescent lights buying my latest three-quarter-length pants – I would look away in horror. Was that me? Really? Oh God. When did that happen?

That wasn't the worst part either. There was a joke in my family that a meal wasn't over until I'd spilled something on my swirly top. To reach my lips, every forkful had to get past the Rock of Gibraltar that was my chest, and at every meal there was at least one spoonful that didn't survive the perilous crossing from plate to mouth.

Not the worst thing by a long mile. My kids loved going to adventure playgrounds, those castle-shaped wooden mazes with lots of twists and turns and bridges and tunnels. When my step-daughter was young I used to race around after her, diving through the tunnels and running over the bridges. That was at 80 kilos. At 122 kilos, I couldn't run around them after my own two young children. The tunnels were too tight, the twists were too narrow. All I could do was stand at the bottom and watch Russell do the chasing. 'You're not as fun as Dad,' my son once told me at a playground when he was little. He was right. I wasn't.

Nowhere near the worst bit yet. I once went for lunch at a Japanese restaurant that had fixed chairs bolted down at fixed tables. Perhaps they thought their clientele was planning to steal them. I tried to squeeze into a chair at one of the tables and couldn't fit. Luckily no one I knew saw me sucking everything in and trying to squeeze into the seat from a variety of different angles. It was no good; I ate at a bench standing up instead.

Just getting to work was hard. Catching the train, I had to go through a gate barrier that I could barely fit past. At first I would go through sideways. That was okay: a little turn to the left did the job. But when I could no longer do that I had to queue up and wait to go through the large magnetic gate for prams, hoping each time I got to the station that this one gate wasn't broken.

And sex? Are you kidding? Having two children and working and studying had already put a dampener on the bedroom department, but putting on 42 kilos was the nail in the love coffin. I was totally uninterested in anything that involved anyone, even Russell, seeing me naked, not that he ever complained.

Not the worst thing yet, but almost. I couldn't fit my engagement ring and wedding ring on my ring finger anymore. These beautiful rings had been my grandmother's. Her marriage had been long and happy and I treasured them, but now they sat on my chest of drawers. I kept meaning to buy a nice chain so that I could wear them around my neck but I never found the time to do it, perhaps secretly hoping I would soon be able to wear them again. And so there they sat, gathering dust – until I came home from work one day to find my bedroom window had been jimmied and the rings were gone.

Still not the worst thing. I snored. I don't mean a gentle occasional rushing sound as I breathed out, I mean *clear-the-tracks-there's-a-runaway-freight-train-on-its-way*. This was possibly one of the reasons I woke up so tired every morning. I went to a sleep doctor and he sent me to a clinic in a hospital where I spent the night in a bed covered in wires with a mask over my face measuring my breathing. The hospital room was right next to the linen cupboard where the ward staff would stop for a chat every twenty or so minutes as they got a bed ready for a new patient. Looking like something out of a sci-fi movie and constantly having to listen to how all the nurses' weekends had been, I managed to fall asleep at 3am. The sleep study operator woke me up at seven. The prognosis was that I had mild sleep apnoea and restless leg syndrome. And the cure? Lose weight. Easier said than done.

Worst thing? Not even close. Under-boob sweat was a constant summer problem at 95 kilos. But as my weight got even higher it turned into a permanent fungal infection that I couldn't get rid of. It was awful and it smelled, making me paranoid about standing close to people. I showered a lot and used a fungal cream that would almost get rid of it, then when I couldn't stand the cream anymore (have you ever tried to wear cream under your bra every day?) I would stop it for a time and the infection would come straight back. Nice.

All the embarrassment and discomfort and bad sleep were awful, but there were also things I was frightened of. I love a long hot bath. Once a week I like to soak off the seven days that have just passed and get ready for the next. But I started to get to the point where I couldn't get out of the bath. Having two children and abdominal surgery for my cancer meant that my stomach muscles had packed their bags, never to return. That was okay; I could still move around, work and study. But the few muscles that were left behind couldn't lift 122 kilos. I had to roll onto my knees and try to get out of the bath that way. Have you ever tried to roll over in a slippery bath? When you already take up most of the room in it? Even when I finally managed to get onto my hands and knees, standing up on a smooth wet surface was hard. One night I slipped and grabbed the edge just in time before I fell. I knew my Sunday bath nights were over.

Have we discussed skin tags yet? Oh, let's do! Skin tags are benign skin tumours, raised from the skin on fleshy peduncles. A 'peduncle' – there's a lovely word to add to my vocabulary of obesity – is a stalk of flesh on which the skin tag grows. A skin tag is like a little eruption of skin. They occur in middle-aged obese people and tend to hang out in places where your skin rubs together. For me that was in my armpits and on my inner thighs. I was so in denial about my body – helped by not having a good-sized mirror in the house – I didn't even notice them when they first appeared.

I like to think of peduncles as spots where my skin just gave up. Like when the *USS Enterprise* is moments away from being sucked into a black hole and Captain Kirk is yelling at Scotty to give him more power and Scotty shouts back, 'I'm giving her all she's got, Captain!' but at the last second finds a little more to save the day. Skin tags were my body saying, 'I'm giving her all she's got, Captain! I can't hold this fat back anymore!' My 130-kilo dad used to get them. Mum would loop a piece of nylon around them and then tie it tight; they would go black and drop off. One of my sisters also got them and had them burned off by her doctor. Over at my place, in denial land, I just ignored them.

I said before that at 122 kilos I could move around okay. That's not exactly true. The skin tags don't make going for a brisk walk easy, but even gentle walking was getting to be hard because of friction. When I was a twenty-two-year-old drama student, still pretty skinny and thinking I was over my teenage puppy-fat phase forever, I was on a tram with an overweight friend when we realised we were going in the wrong direction and had to jump off suddenly. We both stood there watching our tram disappear.

'Let's just walk to the party,' I said. 'It's getting late and it's only one more stop.'

She looked at me nervously, then said, 'Another tram will be along soon.' We both looked down the track. There wasn't another tram in sight.

'It'll only take ten minutes,' I said.

She looked at the ground and blushed. 'I can't,' she said. 'There's friction.'

So, we stood in the cold and waited twenty minutes for the next tram.

Now, sadly, I knew what she meant. There bloody well was friction! At 122 kilos, a half-hour walk around a shopping centre would leave me with a rash on my inner thighs. Another good reason not to exercise. It would go away with some cream and rest. But I knew if I got any heavier it would become permanent, and walking anywhere for any length of time would be a huge problem.

So, was friction the most humiliating thing of all? Was it the pinnacle of my misery? No. The very worst thing was something so awful that if you're squeamish you might want to skip this bit. Seriously, go and make a cup of tea and then flip over to the next page.

At my heaviest I couldn't wipe my own arse. There you have it. Going to the toilet involved contortions of the kind you see only in an advanced yoga class. I once put my back out in the shower doing one of my freaky twists. Do you know that episode of *The Simpsons* where Homer puts on lots of weight so he can work from home? His son, Bart, plans to emulate him when he grows up and has a dream about being hugely obese and TV crews coming to interview him. He tells them, 'I wash myself with a rag on a stick,' and the press take pictures and applaud as he holds up his stick.

I could still manage important daily hygiene procedures with twists and turns and a lot of sucking in, but another few kilos would have done it. What would I have done then? Rag on a stick, I guess.

The rag-on-a-stick threat was a great incentive to lose weight, so it seemed bizarre that after losing 20 kilos and finally being able to give away all my swirly tops and buy normal clothes, I had just gone on a three-day food bender. Had I learned nothing? Keen to understand why I had done it so that it would never happen again, I sat down and mapped out that three-day binge step by step.

I wrote about how I had been travelling to yet another funeral for an uncle. My mother's brother had been overweight and succumbed to a heart problem, and it felt like my small family of large people was leaving us way too fast. I had a grand plan to manage what I ate while away from home. What was it, you ask? I was going to eat lunch when the plane landed at the airport. That was my plan. Eat at the airport. Because airports have such healthy food, don't they? The plane was late leaving, so I had to eat on board, where they served meat pies, sandwiches, chocolates and chips. There was nothing gluten-free except for a chocolate muffin, so I chose something with wheat in it. A chicken tortilla. I didn't want to go to the funeral on an empty stomach.

The funeral service was beautiful. My aunt and two cousins and their partners had put together a very special tribute, and we watched a slide show of my uncle's life. The funeral parlour was packed with his friends and colleagues and it was wonderful to be reminded of how loved he was. All too soon, though, it was late afternoon and time to fly back. I said goodbye and headed to the airport, where my plane was delayed again and I had an hour's wait, which meant I would have to eat there. That was okay, I reassured myself, I could go to the hamburger joint and have a hamburger patty without the bun. But of course the hamburger place was full and instead I went to the Chinese restaurant and chose a bowl of Char Kway Chow with rice noodles. The sticky wheatie oyster sauce on the rice noodles was insanely sweet. After almost four months off sugar, eating those noodles was like eating a bowl of dessert, but I ate it anyway. I was emotional, tired and hungry.

By the time I got home I was even more tired and was now having a huge wheat and sugar freakout. All the old cravings came rushing back. Resisting them felt impossible. It's just one day, I told myself. It's been a difficult day, a very sad day, I deserve this. Then I had a peanut-butter-on-toast festival.

I woke up the next morning craving bread and chocolate. My brain was screaming for it. Screaming. I fought it all day, reminding myself how far I had come, telling myself that I had lost 20 kilos, that fourteen months after not being able to get the seatbelt on the plane around my stomach I had just fitted into one easily, with room to spare. That I could do this, *was* doing this. And then I had the peanut-butter-on-toast festival all over again.

By day three the cravings were just as bad but now I was angry with myself and depressed at my failure. So, I went crazy all day. Ice-cream, biscuits, corn chips.

Luckily on Monday I stopped. I weighed myself first thing in the morning and I had put on 2 kilos – 2 *kilos*! In three days! Luckily I would be seeing Aprille on Friday and therefore had five days of full-time work to help get me back into the rhythm of eating well. I got back to my eating plan and day by day the cravings lessened.

I used the marshmallow experiment to keep myself on track. (And no, I don't mean I ate lots of marshmallows.) This was an experiment first done in the 1970s by a professor at Stanford University. He put four-year-olds one-at-a-time in an empty room with no distractions and then put a marshmallow or a pretzel or a mint on the table in front of them. He explained to the children that they could eat the treat straightaway or wait fifteen minutes and get two. The children who failed to wait often sat and stared at the treat, sometimes even stroking it lovingly. The ones who succeeded in waiting moved to another part of the room, turned away from the marshmallow and distracted themselves by singing a song or playing a game on their fingers or toes. Of course this experiment says a lot about how much trust each child had in authority and whether they actually believed or understood that a second marshmallow would be forthcoming. But it did show that some children had an innate ability to delay gratification, and that their techniques could be copied. The cravings were bad that week but I used a lot of distraction to help deal with them. I wrote in the mornings, I cleaned the house, I went out in the evenings, I worked like a demon at my job during the day.

As the week progressed the cravings lessened, and I learned something really important from that binge. I can't touch wheat or sugar. Ever. Not a grain. Not a speck. Both flip that switch in my head and bring the cravings back instantly. I still have cravings now but they are manageable when I am 100 per cent free of those triggers. That is the number one difference between this way of eating and all the other diets I have been on. The cravings for food are still there but they are quieter. Imagine if you had a voice shouting in your head all the time saying, 'Eat food, eat now, you'll feel better with food, you deserve it, you're hopeless, you'll cope better if you eat something, eat something sweet, eat that pastry, pasta will make you feel better, come on just do it.' Do you know how hard it is to ignore that voice? And the longer you are on a calorie-restricted diet the louder that voice gets as your brain decides you are starving and switches on its battery of hunger hormones to make you eat.

The only option left to me after this was stomach stapling. I've looked into it, even watched TV shows about it. But the idea of clamping off a perfectly healthy organ seems wrong to me. Gastric Bypass (as it is called) patients lose weight because they are starving. They have to take a huge array of nutritional supplements for the rest of their lives to make up for not eating real food and risk many side effects, including death. Plus I've had enough people messing with my insides and would much rather treat the real cause to my weight problem.

And the binge made me think of something else. Could I be scared of losing weight? Of actually succeeding? How else to explain why I sabotaged myself just as I had got under 100 kilos? Was I frightened of being thin? Did this layer of blubber protect me in some way? Was I scared of no longer being the fat invisible middle-aged woman?

It wasn't as if I was waiting until I got thin to start my life. I didn't have all that baggage associated with diets like I did when I was a teenager: of thinking that when I lost weight I would be happy and successful and follow my dreams. I was following my dreams already.

I came across an article that said that obese people make themselves large so that they can take up more space. That they don't have large lives, so they try to make themselves big with their size. Was I afraid of being smaller? Of taking up less space? But no one, especially me, wanted to be obese. That was like saying that people with diabetes who have limbs amputated because of this disease get their diabetes in the first place because they want to be smaller.

What else could I be afraid of? Of having no excuses to not be a lazy parent and to leave all the ball throwing and park visits to my husband? Of having to be strict with what I ate for the rest of my life? Was I afraid of not being the fat funny chick? The fat friend? The fat one in the group? Was I afraid of losing my identity? Was I afraid of all the excess skin I would be left with when I lost weight? Or of being attractive? Was I afraid of having sex with my husband?

Oh hello. Suddenly I had knots in my stomach. I didn't want to think about it. I didn't want to go THERE.

THERE was sexuality. THERE was messed up.

Sex with my husband waned after our first child came on the scene. I had put on a lot of weight and was really tired and stressed and not coping. All good reasons to not be in the mood. Before kids we had a great sex life. And then, after our second child, there was my cancer, and then his cancer. I just wasn't interested in sex anymore and my obesity was my excuse. He never pressured me and we were still very affectionate, hugging, kissing and cuddling. But every now and again I would feel the need to explain to him why I wasn't interested. I would blame it on my weight, but it was more than that. So much more.

My first kiss was in my last year of primary school. I was at a birthday party in Singapore and we played spin the bottle. The bottle stopped at me and I had to kiss a boy with braces. I had braces too and my best friend laughed as we kissed and said, 'Don't get stuck like that forever,' and everyone laughed at us.

A few years later I became close to a boy in Singapore. He was fourteen and I was twelve, and we used to play a fun and very tactile wrestling game in the swimming pool at our apartment where I would have to swim from one side of the pool to the other. To do this I had to get past him standing in the middle, which involved a very long physical wrestling match in the water that he usually won. Then he started kissing me. The wrestling and the kisses all ended the evening his mother came storming down from their apartment and told him to 'Get away from that girl! Your father and I have already warned you. Everyone in the building can see what you are doing!'

What were we doing? It was a game. How come I was suddenly 'that girl'? He didn't say anything to defend me, even though he had started it. I looked up at the twenty-four floors of the apartment building and it felt as if a hundred eyes were watching me. I skulked off home and didn't see the other kids for ages. Being my family, I didn't have anyone I could talk to about all these shameful mixed-up feelings.

My friends at school were all getting into boys and my so-called best friend – the one who laughed at me kissing the boy with braces – kept hassling me to tell her which boy I liked. I was a tomboy and a late bloomer and I didn't like any of them, not in that way, so I just named an innocuous boy whom I knew she wouldn't be interested in. That afternoon she told everyone I liked him.

Then I left Singapore, came back to Melbourne and got fat. Not hugely fat, just plump. Boys, it seems, do not like plump girls. We had to do ballroom dancing in Year 9 and none of the boys from our brother school ever picked me to dance. Pity, because my dad had taught me and I was the only girl in the room who could waltz. One boy did pick me once, when there were more boys than girls and I was the only girl left. He could waltz too. The other couples were stomping around slowly and we moved out of the plodding circle and span around the outside of the ring until the music stopped. It felt great, but he never chose me again.

Then one night, when I was fifteen, I went to a disco in a church hall with some girls from school. I had just finished another huge crash diet and had lost a lot of weight. I was earning a bit of money feeding a dog for a local family who went away on holidays often, and I remember being so hungry on that diet that sometimes I was tempted to eat the dog's food as I spooned it out. At the party a boy started chatting to me and when I said I needed some fresh air he quickly offered to come with me. We walked to a park and kissed. He grabbed my breasts and then tried to put his hand into my underpants, but I stopped him and he took me back to the party. We laughed and joked around some more there until my friend's mum arrived to take us home.

Weeks passed and I heard through a friend that he wanted to see me again. The problem was that I had gone off my diet. My eating was out of control and I had put on weight. A lot of weight. When the same friend organised for a big group of us to go to the movies, he ignored me the whole time. Of course I didn't talk to anyone about this. I wasn't close to my sisters and we weren't encouraged to talk about things at home, plus I didn't have any close friends, so I just bottled it up, as always.

But someone *was* interested in me. In fact he was always kissing my cheek and patting my knee. My eighty-year-old music teacher. Every Wednesday I would have a clarinet lesson with Pop. Lessons weren't much fun but I loved music and was keen to do well. I didn't really like the clarinet but Pop had now started teaching me the guitar, which I liked much more. He started to ask me to kiss him on the cheek at the end of my half-hour lesson. Then he started patting my knee in time to the music. Then I had to give him a kiss and a hug at the end of the lesson. Then one day, to my horror, he grabbed my right breast during our end-of-class hug.

The counsellor I saw after my cancer helped me to see that he had been grooming me all along. Paedophiles pick their targets carefully: kids who won't speak out or who have no one to help them. I wish I had marched straight to the nearest police station after that lesson, but I didn't. At first I thought it had been a mistake. I was fat and unattractive, so why would he have groped me? Or had I led him on? The knee patting had made me feel uncomfortable, but I hadn't known what to do or say to stop it. I didn't want to offend him.

I did do something. I begged my mother to come to my next lesson. 'Come and hear me play. Come and see how good I've got.' It was in the lead up to Christmas and she came grudgingly. He got the message and never touched me again. At the end of the term I dropped out of his classes and completely lost interest in music until I started singing lessons in my thirties. I never did go to the police. He would be long dead now, but I do wonder about who else he had groomed. He was in a small room with the door closed with so many children over the years. Was there anyone else?

And then of course there was my first real boyfriend. I was twenty and had just moved out of home. There were lots of lovely boys, and I was thin and confident on the outside; I had short orange (yes, orange) hair and wore fifties dresses and black lace-up boots. And whom did I choose? The man who did the classic love trap on me. The man who confessed his never-ending love, showered me with flowers and compliments and adoration for about three weeks and as soon as I fell for it pulled all the love away so that I spent a year chasing after it. And he always made me think it was all my fault that he didn't care for me anymore. I was too needy, too fat, too boring, too unadventurous in bed. When I finally saw sense and got out, I was a mess. My fragile, newly earned self-confidence was shot.

Through all these encounters ran a theme: I never felt in control. I always felt as if sex was something done to me, not with me. Even with really lovely boys, during lovemaking I felt as if I were outside of my body watching myself in a movie. Making noises and faces and doing things that I thought I was supposed to be doing. The only person I ever really enjoyed having sex with was Russell. I felt so safe with him, and loved, and cherished.

So, why didn't I want to have sex with him anymore? I knew I needed to face whatever was holding me back, and one morning, lying in bed wrapped together like spoons, I let my hands wander. It's none of your business where they wandered to but my lovely husband didn't get the message until they had well and truly found their mark. I was very nervous, which seems silly after being together for fifteen years, having two children and nursing each other through cancer. He had seen me give birth twice. He had seen every inch of me, thin, fat and even with unspeakable things coming out of both ends of me during one very bad bout of gastro.

And it was lovely. It was as if there hadn't been a gap of several years in our lovemaking. But it was quick.

'Sorry, I'm out of practice,' he said afterwards.

'No problem,' I told him. 'We can spend the rest of our lives practising.' A promise I kept very happily.

So, with the sex problem out of the way, what was stopping me? Was I simply afraid of failing, as I had failed at every other diet I had ever been on? Had I eaten for three days because I was afraid of failing again?

I knew that, whatever the cause, I needed to get back to the plan and keep going. One day at a time. One meal at a time. If I did I would, slowly, slowly, slowly, get there. Surely.

Chapter Seven

99 kilos

I was back under 100 kilos again. No bingeing, no freaking out, no eating at airports. I was sticking to my eating plan and going to the gym once a week. (Once a week isn't great but it's better than nothing.) I was feeling much better and not getting the constant coughs and colds from which I used to suffer. Plus, I was sleeping better. And Russell, although not fat to begin with, had also dropped a few kilos and was looking very svelte.

I flew to Canberra for a writing workshop and the seatbelt fitted even better than the previous flight. No part of my eating plan on that four-day trip involved, 'I'll just grab something at the airport.' I took a truck load of Tupperware and all my food for the first day. I booked a hotel room with a little kitchen and did a supermarket shop as soon as I arrived.

The plane ticket I'd booked allowed me only one suitcase weighing a maximum of 23 kilos, but I'd packed so many layers of clothing for the Canberra winter that I had been barely able to lift my bag and had dreaded how much I'd have to fork out for extra baggage. Somehow I had hauled my suitcase through the airport and hoisted it up onto the scales to find that it weighed 14 kilos. Really? But I'd lost 23 kilos – almost double my suitcase. Suddenly it hit me that I had lost a huge amount of weight.

Feeling pretty happy with myself, I switched on the TV in my room as I was unpacking my groceries. A pygmy hippo at Melbourne Zoo had just given birth to a baby pygmy hippo. The reporter said they didn't know how much the baby hippo weighed yet because the mother and her bub were still in the isolation birthing suite, but that the mother weighed 250 kilos. Excellent. At my heaviest I had weighed half a hippo. Half a pygmy hippo, but still half a hippo. That was a good reason to keep going.

I was still obese; I wouldn't hit the magic 'overweight' category until I was 87 kilos. But even though I was still obese I had done so much for my health and longevity. And it wasn't about how I looked. It wasn't about walking into a room and having every straight man and gay woman go, 'Wow! She's hot!' I was forty-eight. I had two children. This was about being around for them for a very long time. This was about not getting cancer again.

One of the things that started me on this weight-loss mission was an article I read in a magazine when I was 122 kilos. It was by a medical doctor and writer whose writing I really liked, and I eagerly read it to find out whether she had any good medical advice about losing weight. It turned out to be an article implying that fat people must be stupid and that doctors didn't know what to do with them – oh, and how we were responsible for a lot of the world's ills by using up so much of the food resources the planet produced.

The article did discuss the health risks of being overweight or obese, none of which were new to me, such as an increased risk of developing type 2 diabetes, heart disease or of having a stroke, getting gall bladder disease and some cancers – but the sobering part was the disgust she seemed to have for obese people. She began the article with an anecdote – a joke – about an obese woman she stayed with when she was an exchange student and how revolting the woman's eating habits were. It is so easy to make fun of fat people; it doesn't help educate us or change our behaviour.

The worrying thing about the article was that the doctor worked in an obesity clinic. How could she help obese people if she didn't understand them? Imagine if the approach to getting people to stop smoking involved telling them they were just plain stupid and needed more willpower? Smokers are treated like addicts, not idiots. And yet over and over fat people are thought of as stupid or lazy or both. The article stated that being thin was 'a triumph of will over gluttony', and yet we are addicts, just like smokers and drinkers and drug takers. But unlike other addicts we can't go cold turkey. And not only that, we live in a world where everywhere we go we are encouraged to eat, and to eat badly. Every magazine we read, ad break we watch on TV, billboard we go past tells us to eat more processed food and that we will be happy and successful and popular if we do.

Imagine if drugs were legal. Imagine if there were TV ads with football players or top cricketers saying, 'I eat eight blocks of crack for breakfast. How many can you eat?' Or signs on the freeway asking if we'd shot up today? This is what obese people have to deal with constantly. Is it any wonder we give in? So much needs to change if we are going to tackle the obesity crisis, not least people's disgust for the overweight.

I was on a ferry once, with my son when he was quite little. We were going for a ride up the Yarra River on a sunny day and the crew included a large young woman in her twenties. As she wound ropes and readied the ferry to depart, a family got on – grandparents, their children and grandchildren – who were all slim. They sat down and the adults started making cruel fat jokes about the woman, in front of the children. Having to hear their sneering was awful, but I had my revenge: I didn't tell them they were on the wrong boat.

I'm sure people have talked about me behind my back. I just don't like to think about it. When my sister Ruth went to Vietnam she kept hearing people say, 'Đít bự,' as she walked past. She found out later it meant 'big arse'.

When I see someone really overweight I want to go up to them, take their hand and say, 'Wheat and sugar. Stop eating them both. You don't have a laziness problem. You have an appetite problem. You have an insulin problem.' But I don't. That would humiliate them. I just hope that somehow they find the support and skills to find out for themselves.

Interestingly, just after I got back from Canberra the same medical writer published a follow-up article. She discussed how she had been attacked by the 'fat is beautiful' lobby for her first article but how she still stood her ground in saying that fat wasn't beautiful; that it was a dangerous health condition. This time she dropped the fat jokes and the sneering, which was a much better approach. I agreed with her 100 per cent.

I understand where the 'fat is beautiful' lobby comes from. It's not fair that women have to be dangerously thin to be considered beautiful. And that what would have been considered beautiful fifty years ago is now considered fat. It also sucks that being overweight destroys your self-esteem just when you need it most to love yourself and eat well.

But I stand firmly with the medical journalist in the 'obesity is really dangerous' camp. Wrapping your organs in tentacles of subcutaneous fat makes you very sick and you will die much earlier than you should. It's as simple as that. In her second article she still didn't have any good answers to how the health profession can help obese people. But we do agree on one thing: obesity kills. And that's not attractive on any level.

So, now I was under 100 kilos. My weight-loss journey was going slowly but well. I had Aprille and Mischa. I had a routine. I was focused. But life was about to throw me another curve ball. And I didn't see it coming.

Chapter Eight

98 kilos

It was 11.30am on a Wednesday and I was at work. I was talking to one of my lovely interns when suddenly a wave of panic hit me from nowhere. A tsunami of fear. I breathed and concentrated on what we were talking about, but another one came. And another. If my terror meter went from one to ten, this was a twenty. I wasn't just frightened. I was frightened I was going to die. Not die exactly – it felt as if the world was suddenly tilting and I was going to fall off and keep falling forever.

I managed to mumble something about going for a walk to my intern, grabbed my bag and coat and stumbled outside. I stood on the street shaking. I had never had an attack so bad that I had to leave work. Never. I hadn't had an attack this bad since my cancer.

My arms and legs were shaking, everything looked too close up, and sounds were loud and intrusive. I knew this was all part of the fight-or-flight reflex. When you have a panic attack your body floods with adrenaline and in response the brain transfers blood from your digestive system and other organs to your arms, legs, sight and hearing. This all happens in a split second so you can turn and fight the charging lion or run from it.

But I had no lion. All I had was a too-bright city street with crowds of people going about their busy day while my life crumbled.

I didn't know what to do. Should I go home? Go back to work and tough it out? I couldn't call Russell as he was at work plus my instinct, as always, was to try and sort it out myself. I started walking as waves of terror crashed on top of me relentlessly. I tried to do my self-talk: *These are just thoughts, I told myself. They can't hurt you. This isn't real. You are fine.* It didn't help.

One sane thought crashed through. *I need food.* I stumbled into a petrol station and didn't know what to buy. The shelves swam in front of me and I couldn't focus. I grabbed a Mars Bar, paid and ate it as I kept walking. I made it to a park on the edge of the city, where I found a seat and slumped down. I thought sitting in nature might help but it didn't, and as soon as I stopped walking another massive wave swept over me.

I kept walking and circled slowly back to work. *I'll just go inside, I told myself, to say I don't feel well. Then I'll go home. But what if I can never go back to work again? What if I am like this forever?*

I got back to work and started talking again to my intern, trying to regain my composure. Then a writer dropped in with some questions and I got caught up in the moment and the busyness of the office and before I knew it, it was 5.30pm. Home time. Thank God.

I made it home but I was jittery and tense. And of course I didn't tell anyone what was happening, not even Russell.

Anxiety is so internal. If you were sitting right next to me during an attack you wouldn't know it. You might just notice that I had gone a bit quiet.

I didn't sleep well and went to work the next day dreading it happening again. And it did. I didn't leave this time but had to manage hours of panic all day. Again it was the falling-off-the-end-of-the-world-into-a-void-of-nothingness panic. But 5.30pm blessedly arrived again and I had made it through. Friday was a repeat of Wednesday and Thursday.

I thought the weekend would help. That I would relax and be able to step back from this cliff-edge tension that was gripping me day and night. That I would sleep and by Monday I would be over the worst. I had stopped taking my anxiety medication because things had been so good lately. I started back on it and upped the dose to 100mg from my usual 50mg.

But the weekend was awful. I couldn't relax. I woke up on Saturday and Sunday straight into the shock of being immediately swamped with fear. On Sunday night I had five hours of straight panic. One wave of terror after another. I paced the house all night. I thought very seriously about driving myself to a psychiatric hospital and begging them to knock me out with drugs just to stop it. I finally fell into a sleep from exhaustion. I woke up and the panic was instantly in my face.

My panic is a very private thing: I never, ever talk about it. My best friends don't know about it. It is something I feel very ashamed of, and besides, talking about it makes it real. When I am okay I feel silly about being such a slave to these stupid thoughts. It was just something I managed.

But I couldn't manage this alone. So, I told Russell. He was surprised. Because I never talk about it he doesn't know what a big part of my life managing it is. And then I had to call work. I started crying before our director even answered her phone. I managed to gulp out what was happening, and she very sweetly told me to take some time off, get some help and that when I had a plan, to call her back and let her know what it was.

A plan. I needed a plan. I called my counsellor, Jenny, the one I had seen when Russell was ill. She had been marvellous through that difficult time. Her receptionist told me they had just had a cancellation and Jenny could see me the next day. I relaxed for a moment and then the fear came flooding back.

I made it through the next twenty-four hours and when I saw Jenny we talked about how I needed to see a psychiatrist, how I needed to sort out my medication and that my GP wouldn't be able to do that. She knew a good one who was new to the area so might be able to fit me in soon. I called him when I got home and, like Jenny, he told me he'd just had a cancellation and could fit me in the next day. The universe was being extra good to me. I could make it through one more day.

The psychiatrist's name was Ben. He charged $365 for a one-hour consultation. Luckily we still had money from the sale of my house and I would also get a big chunk of his fee back from Medicare. I was about to benefit from the private mental-health system again.

I sat nervously in the waiting room – well, extra nervously because I did everything nervously now. What if he told me I was crazy? What if he told me I would never work again? Or worst of all – what if there was absolutely nothing he could do to help me and I was going to feel like this forever?

He came out and smiled at me. A big, warm smile. Then he showed me to his room, where on his desk sat a big plastic replica of an abdomen. 'This is the room for the bariatric surgery patients,' he explained when he saw me looking at the clamped-off stomach. Ironic. Oh, if only I was there for weight loss.

I told him what had been happening, how my increase in anxiety had been sudden and severe. I asked him if I was going crazy.

He smiled again. 'I work at a big public hospital as the emergency-room psychiatrist. I see an awful lot of very ill people. Trust me, you're not crazy.'

I relaxed, not much but as much as I was able to at that moment. I told Dr Ben about how life was good – really good – and I couldn't understand why I had anxiety now. He delved a little deeper into my recent past and I told him about how two years ago Russell had been diagnosed with secondary skin cancer and suffered psychosis. He diagnosed me with Post Traumatic Stress Disorder.

Post Traumatic Stress Disorder? That didn't seem right. I had coped so well with Russell's illness and now I was falling apart? I told a friend who was a psychologist and she said, 'Oh yes, we get that at the clinic all the time. People come in and say, "Life's good but I've fallen apart." Then you dig into their history and hear that two years ago they had an awful car accident or illness or lost a loved one. Two years. You can set your watch by it.'

So, Dr Ben was right. Somehow having the label of PTSD didn't make me feel like such an idiot. Dr Ben put my medication up to 150mg and I started seeing Jenny once a week. I also went back to all the things that had helped me when my anxiety had gone off the scale after my cancer seven years ago. I didn't rest or sit with the anxiety. I kept moving. Pottering. Hanging out clothes. Doing dishes. Sweeping the leaves from the driveway; our driveway never looked so good. I couldn't watch most TV shows but I did find one that I could: *Family Feud*. It had nothing scary or upsetting or too dramatic in it. Whenever I got too tired to do housework or sweep I would watch an episode. Grant Denyer, the host, and his daggy sense of humour saved me. In the show contestants are asked a question and have to match the top answers that 100 random people have given. Grant would do accents or silly dances and sometimes I would almost laugh.

I would sit and watch, answering the questions and getting most of them wrong. The increased medication made me fuzzy and affected my short-term memory. Sometimes I would be halfway through an episode, getting all the answers right for a change, when I would realise I had watched it already. Name something you might see on a golf course was one of the questions. Goats was the answer given. Not surprisingly, a hundred random people had not listed goats as their top answer. The top answer was golfers.

Name when this anxiety is going to stop? No answer for that one.

After two weeks off work I felt a bit better. Dr Ben had put me on sleeping pills, which I had umm-ed and ahh-ed about taking, remembering how I had been hooked on them in my early twenties, but Dr Ben smiled and said, 'You don't actually have a choice.' He was right. I didn't. The ones he gave me weren't addic-tive. I took my first one, slept till 10am the next day, then snoozed on the couch all the rest of the day.

But I couldn't stay at home snoozing and watching *Family Feud* for the rest of my life. Both of my kids were at school and I had to go back to work. I knew from past experience that if you keep avoiding things that are hard, anxiety can shrink your world very quickly until you live in a small bubble of your home and a few local places you aren't afraid to go to.

I called work and they were supportive and flexible, and agreed to my coming back on reduced hours. Our Director, Kate, and our

General Manager, Jac, said that if I ever needed to leave to just tell them and go, and that my reduced hours could be for as long as I needed. What wonderful bosses. I counted my blessings again for having such a fantastic job.

On my first day back I stood at the train station trying to breathe and telling myself everything was okay. I had worked at Writers Victoria for a year and a half, and made this trip countless times. I would be fine. I managed to catch the train and get to work. I arrived with my legs shaking, and although I tried to joke around and act normal, inside I was a mess. My vision would blur and swim and my heart would race. But I made it through the first day. Just five hours, but it seemed like forever.

I was doing only fifteen hours a week. The mornings were the worst: rolling panic for three hours. Somehow after lunch I would be better. Maybe the food helped or maybe my brain was just too damn tired to think of anything at all – scary or otherwise – in the afternoon. With my short-term memory still affected I had to check everything I did several times, but I managed to get by and to not muck too many things up. And I got back to class, shaking, trying to hide my fear and praying that no one would workshop any writing that was too dark or frightening. I would drive to class and park close by so I had a quick escape route, which is ironic because there is no escape from anxiety.

Jenny convinced me that I wasn't going to fall off the end of the world and keep falling. 'You've had the worst of the anxiety. This is as bad as it's going to get. And you coped.'

She was right. My Richter Scale of panic wasn't going to get any higher. This idea helped calm me down a bit, enough to sometimes do a whole day at work. Weeks passed and I was managing work and study but still not really improving much more. Dr Ben put my medication up to 200mg.

'When will it kick in?' I kept asking him.

'Give it time,' he said. 'This anxiety has built up over two years; it's not going to go away overnight.'

Had it been building for two years? Jenny and I started to look back. We discovered that my attacks had been getting steadily worse over the past six months and I had been ignoring them. Things I had been used to doing, like going to writing events and forums, had become hard and I had stopped pushing myself to go to them. My world had started to shrink and I hadn't paid attention to it. I had got into a manuscript-development and publishing program in Canberra and had had a monster attack in my hotel room at the first workshop, but had still thought it was a good idea to go off my medication only a few months later. That attack had been a big warning sign that I had ignored. I was a ticking time bomb. I still hadn't processed a lot of the distress of Russell's illness, I wasn't doing things to help my anxiety, like being mindful and watching my self-talk, and to top things off I had been playing with my medication. Plus, I had been pushing myself hard: full-time work, study, the Canberra program, working on my detective novel plus raising two school-aged children. And I had been really ill twice that year and hadn't seen it as a sign that I had taken on too much and was getting worn down.

So, I accepted that this was going to take a while and tried to be gentle on myself. And the kids were happy to play endless board games with me in my effort to stay focused and in the moment. One other thing I did that I had never done before was to tell people what was happening. I had told a few very close friends about my anxiety after my cancer but I had never raised it again. Now I told people at work and I told some friends. I told my writing group and when I asked to have a meeting at my house they didn't ask questions. And when the second Canberra workshop came up and I couldn't go I told the other writers in the program. It felt scary and liberating to be so open. Others shared their history with anxiety with me and it helped to know it was so common.

With all these steps I should have been getting better, but I wasn't. I got grumpy with Dr Ben. 'You said I'd be okay to go to Canberra for the second writing workshop and I wasn't. I couldn't go. When am I going to get better?'

'Give it time,' he assured me.

'I don't know how much more of this I can take,' I admitted.

Anxiety wears you down, bit by bit. I was still waking up and instantly being swamped with it, I was still shaking at work and struggling through each day. There was no light at the end of my dark tunnel. Last time I had severe anxiety, the medication had fixed it. But now I was up to 200mg, the highest recommended dose, and it still hadn't kicked in.

'Vigorous exercise.'

I looked at Dr Ben. Did he just say exercise? I was paying him $255 for a half-hour session every week and all he had was exercise?

'I tried exercise after my cancer. I walked for forty minutes every day without fail and it didn't help my anxiety.'

'Not gentle exercise. Vigorous exercise. You have to sweat.'

I hate to sweat. 'What about a different medication? There are other types. Can't we try a different one?'

Dr Ben smiled. 'The thing about another medication is that it will only have a 30 to 50 per cent chance of working. And we know your current medication works. It's worked before. Just give it time. And try vigorous exercise.'

I left wondering if I could get in to see another psychiatrist. But then I thought about the six-week wait and also that I should give 'vigorous exercise' a try before telling Dr Ben at next week's appointment that it was rubbish.

That night I played badminton with my son for an hour at a local indoor centre. I played hard. I played till I couldn't breathe. I played till I almost won a game off him. The next day I worked from 9.30am till 5.30pm with no anxiety.

Sorry, Dr Ben, you were right.

As soon as I came home from work I put on my sneakers and ran. And ran. And ran. The first night I ran 2 kilometres without stopping, panting, 'I can beat this,' with every step. Not my old shuffling-type half-running, but real running. Badminton, gym, personal training, laps and laps of the local pool. I did something 'vigorous' every day. Something that had me red-faced with sweat pouring off my nose. Anything to keep the anxiety at bay. And it worked.

Jenny and Dr Ben explained what was happening. When you have an attack your body floods with adrenaline. I knew that but what I didn't know was that the adrenaline can take ten days to drain away. Ten days! So, if you have several attacks each day the adrenaline never drains. It just keeps building up causing more anxiety, which results in more adrenaline, which results in more anxiety. A vicious cycle that is heavy on the vicious.

'It's a miracle!' I told Dr Ben. He just smiled.

I was able to work three full days a week and take a train to my writing class with no problems. I could watch proper TV. I could read. My anxiety was still a bit elevated but I was out of the crisis period. I knew because I suddenly had hope that I would eventually return to normal – and when things had been bad I didn't have hope. Hope is the difference between crisis and recovery. When you cross that line and feel hope again it is wonderful.

You know that sliver of good? Yes, there's one in this situation too. Severe anxiety is really good for weight loss, and the next 8 kilos fell off me. I am not encouraging people who want to lose weight to develop an anxiety disorder – I wouldn't wish anxiety on my worst enemy – I'm just saying it had a benefit. My appetite was down and I stopped snacking and I was exercising hard every day. I stuck to my meal plan and the kilos melted away.

That's the great thing about this way of eating. If you overeat you don't do too much damage. If you binge on nuts and cheese you only put on a small amount. How much you lose and how quickly is just a matter of fine-tuning your portion sizes and your snacking. I could have lost weight at this dramatic rate all along if I had been really tough on myself. The reason it had taken me sixteen months to lose 30 kilos was that I refused to ever starve. Flat-out refused. And you don't have to starve when you eat this way.

So, there I was, 92.8 kilos. A BMI of 32. There was something I could do now. Something I had wanted to do for a long time.

It was time to have my boobs cut off.

Chapter Nine

92 kilos

I wanted to go back to the Arsehole Surgeon and say, 'Ta da! I did it.' But he charged $200 for a consultation and I didn't really want to pay that much money to rub his face in my weight loss, so I looked online for another surgeon. I found one who had published papers and sat on training boards, and had lots of glowing online testimonials. He was so busy I couldn't get in to see him for six weeks, which I took as a very good sign.

On the day of the appointment Mr Dean examined me thoroughly and took my measurements. I noticed he had thank-you cards along his window ledge.

'How attached are you to your belly button?' he said.

'Excuse me?'

Mr Dean explained. 'There are some risks with any surgery, but with this surgery one of the small risks is that I may not be able to re-attach your belly button.'

Time to fess up. I wasn't just talking to Mr Dean about having a breast reduction, I was also chatting to him about a tummy tuck. Yes, I know that's cheating. But I have a big pannis – another lovely word to add to my obesity vocabulary. A pannis isn't something sticky and sweet you buy from a Greek delicatessen. It's a big semicircle of fat and skin that hangs down from your stomach when you lose a lot of weight. Plus, I had a large hernia that my cancer surgeon, Mr Stephen, would prod every year when I saw him for my annual check-up and then would tell me I should do something about. Mr Stephen said that hernias were dangerous and could strangulate my bowel. Plus my insides pushed through the hernia every time I did a sit-up. Not in an *Alien* movie kind of way, just as a weird bump that would appear and disappear with every exertion. So, talking about a tummy tuck wasn't just vanity, it was about important health care . . . and a bit of vanity.

Mr Dean asked me to disrobe down to my undies then he got out his camera and measuring tape. I was still wearing the concrete-bunker bra and it was still fitting me snugly, even though I'd lost 20 kilos since I bought it. Mr Dean took lots of photos of me from different angles and took measurements. The photos weren't for his amusement or his website, they were for training purposes, to help guide his surgery and to show to other patients who were considering the same surgery. (My head would be cut off in all the photos, so my saggy boobs and tummy would be unidentifiable.)

I told him how I had lost 30 kilos but still had gigantic breasts that hadn't shrunk at all. He explained that no matter how much weight I lost it wouldn't affect my breast size too much, and that surgery wouldn't leave me with perfect breasts but would take the weight off my chest, which would make life a lot easier. He showed me before and after photos of patients similar to me whose new breasts looked pretty damn perfect from where I was sitting. My right breast is markedly bigger than the left because I am right-handed, and he explained that he would be able to make my breasts the same size. He asked me if I had a final size in mind and I said no, that I would leave that up to him to give me a size he thought would suit my body shape. His shoulders relaxed. 'I wish every patient would say that,' he told me with a smile.

Then he talked me through the abdominal surgery. He explained that he would do a low cut from hip bone to hip bone, then would repair the hernia, put in mesh to support my abdominal muscles, pull the skin back down, cut off the excess and sew me back up. Doing both operations together would take six hours and I would be off work for about three weeks.

He was so thorough and kind. He even laughed at one of my jokes and made a few of his own before taking me to his office manager to discuss costs. Good thing I was sitting down when she told me I was going to be out of pocket $15,000. I'd stopped making jokes by then. She explained that Medicare regarded each breast as a different surgery, so having a breast reduction and tummy tuck was actually regarded as three different operations. I thought this was outrageous. I mean, who on earth would have surgery on just one breast? Then I realised that women who have breast cancer do just that and that I was lucky to be having this surgery for comfort and lifestyle rather than life-threatening necessity. And that it was cosmetic surgery and that of course I should pay for the bulk of it.

Now, how would I tell Russell? I caught the train back home with all my brochures tucked away in the bottom of my bag. Although I knew Russ was very supportive of the breast reduction, I hadn't mentioned the idea of a tummy tuck to him. How attached was he to what was left of our nest egg?

Lying in bed that night I ran it past him, emphasising the importance of getting my hernia fixed. He was fine with it and I called Mr Dean's office the next day and booked in for the end of April.

Mr Dean had said the results from both operations would be better if I was closer to my final goal weight. I had six months, therefore, to lose as much weight as I could. It was time to get serious about exercise. I had slacked off after my anxiety had reduced and was only going to see Mischa every Sunday for personal training and wasn't doing anything else the rest of the week. My diet was absolutely on track. I wondered if I could speed things up with more exercise. I'd heard about something called interval training where you exercise intensely for a short period of time a few times per week. I didn't like the 'intense' part but the 'short period of time' sounded really good. I hit the web and did a search for HIIT (High Intensity Interval Training) along with the name of my suburb, not expecting any results. The first result was a class nearby three times a week.

I knew it would be good for my lingering anxiety and for getting me in shape for the surgery, so before I could chicken out I booked in. Two days later I was in a local church hall in daggy grey track pants with twenty incredibly fit women all wearing active wear. I looked around, trying to see who the instructor was so I could tell them I was a complete newbie, but any one of those women in neon funky gym gear could be the instructor. I made my way to the back of the hall and waited for the class to start. The only guy in the room leaped onto the stage. Ah, he was the instructor.

'Is anyone new to the class?' he asked.

My hand shot up and he leaped off the stage to come to see me.

'Just do your best and stop at any time if you need to. There's a modified version of each exercise, so choose that one if you need to.'

I nodded. How hard could it be? I'd lost 30 kilos. I'd been going to a personal trainer for eighteen months. I'd be fine.

So. Not. Fine.

After just the five-minute warm-up I was sweating like a pig and panting like a smoker climbing stairs. How many burpees can you fit into one twenty-minute session? A lot, it seems. How many times can you hop and jump and throw yourself on the floor then get straight back up? Also a lot. After the class I drove home with shaking legs and lay my head on the kitchen table and panted for a further ten minutes. It was insane. And everyone but me kept up.

I didn't go back. Not because the class was ridiculously hard (which it was) or because I hated the blaring techno music (which I did) or because I was in track pants and everyone else looked like they had just stepped out of a Lorna Jane brochure, but because I didn't have fun and felt intimidated.

Thirty kilos down and I still wasn't confident enough to mix it with uber-mums in lycra. That Sunday I went to Mischa's, as usual. She was playing R&B soul music, and we talked about writing, because she used to be a journalist and had written two books. I felt comfortable and accepted. I didn't tell her I had tried another class and sheepishly asked if she had heard of HIIT training. She had, of course. She was running a few sessions of it a couple of times a week and I made a commitment to start going to one of her classes. I had finally found my exercise home after years of looking. Going to the super-fit active-wear class had just confirmed that for me.

Summer arrived and with it trips to the nearby beach. Squeezing my huge breasts into my bathers for the first time, I cracked it. I'd had enough. I couldn't wait until the end of April to be rid of them. I phoned Mr Dean's office and said I was desperate and just wanted the breast reduction and not to worry about the tummy tuck at this stage. His office manager said she would speak to him and then called me straight back. They had found a spot six weeks earlier than my scheduled surgery, which gave me three months to lose as much weight as I could. There was only one problem: I was 92 kilos. I knew what that meant. Plateau time!

One of the great things about losing so much weight over a long period is that you get to know your patterns. My pattern is that I plateau every 10 kilos. I had a massive plateau at 112 kilos, another one at 102 kilos and here I was at 92 kilos and the scales wouldn't budge.

But this time around I knew what was happening. I didn't panic. I didn't call myself a hopeless loser or look for reasons I couldn't lose anymore weight. I just went with it. Sometimes the scales would dip and then bounce back up, but I couldn't crack getting under 90 kilos to save my life. And the months ticked by, so I just let them. Aprille was keen to help and suggested lots of tweaks and changes, but I knew I just needed a rest for a while. I never wanted to starve myself ever again and I was happy to cruise in the knowledge that more weight loss would eventually happen.

The only issue was that my surgery was impending and Mr Dean had said the result would be better if I was closer to my goal weight. One week before the surgery Aprille gave me a pep talk.

'You have one week to go, just get under 90 kilos. Cut out the nuts and cheese and the night-time eating. Focus. And text me each morning.'

Back to the texting? Really? But I knew she was right. I said goodbye to macadamias and Jarlsberg, and my body celebrated big time. Apparently it had been ready to end the plateau ages ago. The weight just dropped off me that week. The morning of the surgery I was 87.25 kilos. No longer obese, I was now merely overweight. Not something you would normally celebrate, but I did . . . with a sip of dandelion coffee and a small bowl of my seed cereal. It was 6.45am. From 7am I wasn't allowed to eat or drink anything, even water.

It was surgery day.

Chapter Ten

87 kilos

What do you pack in a suitcase for an overnight stay in hospital for a breast reduction?

Slippers: check. Dressing-gown: check. A book to read: check. Anxiety medication: check. Nightgown: check. Comfy clothes to wear home: erm . . . What size would I be when I went home? Would there be swelling? Bandages? I put in my favourite T-shirt – size 20 – knowing it might be the last time I'd ever wear it.

Russell drove me to the train station and hefted my suitcase out of the trunk of the car. I had insisted that he didn't take the morning off work to drive me to the hospital. He wrapped his arms around me.

'Nervous?'

I nodded vigorously.

'Excited?'

I nodded again.

'You'll be fine.'

We kissed goodbye and I headed off for the platform, more nervous than I had been for my bowel cancer operation. That surgery had been essential; there had been no question of not having it. This was elective surgery. Worse, it was cosmetic elective surgery. What if it went wrong? What if I died? I'd feel pretty stupid then, assuming dead people could feel stupid. Or what if I ended up paralysed or had a stroke or it all went horribly wrong and I had terrible infections and needed more surgery and regretted this for the rest of my short hospitalised life?

You can probably see why I suffer from anxiety. Catastrophising? Oh yes, I have a PhD in it. As the train rocked back and forth I reminded myself how safe this surgery was, how good my surgeon was, how wonderful it would be not to carry two watermelons around on my chest for the rest of my life. I also reminded myself that I had already paid for it. Upfront. In full: $8500. When the train arrived I jumped off and wheeled my ridiculously heavy suitcase to the hospital.

The small bowl of cereal I had eaten seemed like an eon ago and I was starting to feel light-headed. I checked in and joined the other patients waiting to be called. There were a lot of us. Young, old, male, female. I knew I was the only one having a breast reduction, though. None of them, male or female, had watermelons like mine.

There was a big sign saying, 'You will not be called in order of arrival.' The sign didn't lie. More people arrived. I waited and waited. More people trotted off to have their hearing fixed (the shouty man), their knees sorted (the hobbling woman in shorts with a criss-cross of scars on her knee), their cataracts done (the old lady with the misty eyes clinging to her husband). I don't know if any of that is true. I don't actually know why they were there. We didn't chat. We all sat quietly, heads down, the only sound the turning of magazine pages. Except for Shouty Man. We all knew why he was there.

Finally my name was called. I wheeled my suitcase through the magic door but was told to turn right. This was just a pre-op meeting with one of the nurses. My height was taken and I was weighed. 88.4 kilos. Not fair! I had clothes on. And shoes. And I'd had some cereal this morning. I wasn't obese. I offered to take my shoes off and be weighed again but she said it didn't matter. Hell yes it did, but I decided not to argue.

'What are you here for?' she asked.

I thought of making a joke. Something about a bank-account amputation. The cereal had been a really long time ago and I was now very light-headed but I resisted the urge. Now was not the time for jokes, even bad ones.

'Breast reduction.'

'Which breast?'

We looked at my watermelons. 'Both,' I replied, again resisting the urge to joke.

'Good. Always important to make sure we think you are here for the same reason you think you are here.'

Damn. Perhaps I could have slipped in the tummy tuck without having to pay extra.

She clipped a hospital ID to both of my wrists and one to my right leg. Then I was sent back to the waiting room. Now it was just me and Shouty Man and the cross-looking middle-aged business type in the suit. I tried to pick what he was there for. He looked so furious, scowling at his *Financial Review* magazine. Who wears a suit to surgery? Maybe he had come from work. Or maybe he wore a suit everywhere. Maybe on the weekends he played tennis in a suit.

Okay. Very light-headed now.

Shouty Man was called. Then Suit Man was called. It was after 4pm. Finally it was my time. I went through the magic door and was guided to a cubicle with a mirror and a seat with a gown hanging up in it. I was told to take everything off but my undies; to put it all in my suitcase and then put the gown on.

But my suitcase was full. I was beginning to regret bringing so much. With lots of grunting and pushing and sitting on top of it I got my clothes in the suitcase and shut it. Then I took one last look at my droopy watermelons and put the gown on.

I was sent to a small room full of suitcases. And a toilet. And Suit Man in a gown. He looked up and smiled at me. A kind of a good-luck-don't-we-look-stupid smile. He should take off the suit more often, I thought. He looked ten years younger.

Then he was called to go in. Lucky him. And I was alone with the suitcases. Not long after, I was finally called too. I was taken into a huge room with people on trolleys lined up in neat rows. There were quite a few people lying on them waiting to be wheeled through to their surgery. A nurse approached me. She checked my ID tags and showed me which trolley to lie on. It was really good to lie down.

'What are you here for?' she asked.

'A bilateral breast reduction,' I replied. I was learning the lingo. She took my blood pressure then asked me if I had anything in my body that I wasn't born with. I was tempted to say enormous breasts but that wasn't what she meant.

She explained. 'A pacemaker, stents, metal hip implant, piercings?'

I shook my head.

'Nope. This is all me.'

Pretty soon I was wheeled off to another cubicle (hospitals do love their cubicles) just outside an operating theatre, and I was told it wouldn't be long now.

Suddenly I got nervous. Really nervous. Panic-attack nervous. I told myself it was okay to be nervous. And that I hadn't had any food for a long time. And that Mr Dean was an excellent surgeon who could do this operation in his sleep and that in two to three hours it would be over. I told myself how great the results of the surgery would be. I also wished I hadn't been so stoic, telling Russell I could cope all by myself, that it was too far for him to come. I wanted someone's hand to hold.

Luckily, things got busy. The anaesthetist, Dr Craig, came and asked me questions about any previous surgery, medications, my general health. Then he inserted a cannula tube into the vein in my left hand and taped it down. Then Mr Dean arrived, looking tired. He had probably been operating since early morning. He was holding a bunch of permanent markers in different colours and got me to sit up and take off my gown, then started marking my chest. A blue circle here, a black line there, two yellow crosses there. I looked like a road map.

'Not long now,' he said smiling.

He was right. When I had my cancer surgery the operating room had been huge and full of people. This one was quite small. And it had a window, like a treatment room rather than a theatre. I was disappointed at its lack of grandness. It was almost cosy.

'What are you having done today?' Mr Dean asked.

'Bilateral breast reduction,' I said, right on cue.

Mr Dean nodded then Dr Craig injected something into the cannula. 'You'll start to feel relaxed now.'

I don't like drugs. I don't like losing control. But I was so happy to have that warm fuzzy feeling wash through me and to sink into the thin mattress on the operating table. Surgery is actually quite easy, really. You don't have to do anything. You just have to lie there. So, I just lay there as one of the technicians strapped two blue puffy things to my legs.

'You're going to get a nice leg massage while we operate,' he told me. 'To help stop you getting a DVT. That's a deep vein thrombosis.'

Dr Craig leaned over me. 'Ready to go? I've just given you the main anaesthetic.'

'You beschtchas . . .' I said, trying to give him a thumbs-up but not being able to figure out where my thumbs were.

When I had my cancer surgery I remember counting down from ten and only making it to six, then opening my eyes in the recovery room as if no time had passed at all. The operation to remove a third of my bowel had taken three hours.

This time I don't remember being in recovery. I don't remember opening my eyes or being wheeled from recovery to the ward. I remember being moved onto a bed in a darkened ward with curtains drawn around me. And I remember the pain. Oh, the pain. A lovely nurse named Miriel asked me how bad the pain was out of ten. I thought about childbirth and said seven. If you've given birth then you'll know that seven is actually really high on the pain scale.

But I do remember those awful blue puffy things, which were still attached to my legs. Not massaging, like the nurse in the operating theatre had said, but squeezing hard then deflating then inflating and squeezing hard all over again . . . and again . . . and again. I remember trying to shift myself up the bed to get more comfortable and not being able to move because of those wretched blue things and because of the pain. So much pain.

Then it was morning. I hadn't slept much thanks to the pain and the evil blue things. Then breakfast arrived. Miriel put more pillows under my head so I could see the tray of food. On it were cornflakes, two pieces of white toast with a small container of margarine and one of strawberry jam, a bowl of tinned peaches and a glass of orange juice. Nothing I could eat. Not that I felt like eating. Did I mention the pain? Still at a seven.

117

'Do you need to go to the toilet?' asked Miriel.

'Yes.'

'Do you think you could manage walking to the toilet?'

I looked at the three steps it would take to get from my bed to the toilet. 'No.'

So, I lay there on a bedpan, in agony, blue things squeezing my legs and looking at a tray of sugar and wheat.

Suddenly this whole breast-reduction scheme seemed like a really bad idea.

But then I looked down at my chest and finally it was all worth it. I had perky, cute, normal-sized breasts.

I won't bore you with the rest of my hospital stay. The food got much better – poached-salmon-with-a-crust-of-pesto better. The nurses were all amazing, the only hiccup being the male nurse who showered me on my first day putting the compression bra on me backwards; I wore it backwards for a whole week before I realised it was meant to button up in the front. It had a wide back, which is why it kind of sort of looked okay buttoned up wrong.

I ended up staying for two nights. My two sisters visited, and Russ came with our daughter, who went all shy and nervous. She wouldn't hug me and sat on her daddy's knee, biting the corner of her thumb and giving me monosyllabic answers.

'How was school today?'

'Good.'

'How was saxophone?'

'Good.'

'Are you tired, sweetheart?'

'Yes.'

'Do you want to go home?'

'Yes.'

I guess she didn't like the sight of me in a hospital bed.

Mr Dean visited each day. He told me he had taken 2 kilos off my chest: 1.2 kilos off the big right breast and 800 grams off the left. He said the pain would be at its worst for the first twenty-four hours and then would quickly subside. He was right. I was sent home with Panadol. Strong Panadol but Panadol.

At my one-week check-up I mentioned to Mr Dean that I suddenly felt so tall and straight. Two kilos is a lot of weight to carry around on your chest, pulling you down and forwards, constantly hurting your back and neck. Mr Dean told me that one of his nurses actually asked him if their breast-reduction patients do get taller after the surgery, and he had said no, they just stand taller. He was so right.

I had two and a half weeks at home and then returned to work. It was funny being back in the world. Everyone who knew about the surgery looked at my breasts. Not directly, just surreptitiously, out of the corner of their eyes. I got around this by inviting them to have a good look.

'Go ahead. I can't stop staring at them either,' I'd tell them. 'They're pretty awesome.'

And they are. Thanks, Mr Dean and your amazing team.

Chapter Eleven

85 kilos

I was back at the gym. Mischa said I was much lighter on my feet. She had me in the boxing ring now and was constantly correcting my technique.

'Straighten your arms . . . turn your hips . . . you've dropped your hands, you're wide open, keep them up near your chin . . . plant your feet, don't punch from your toes . . .'

I hadn't been doing real boxing until now. I don't mean Mischa had been training me badly, but I think she had been focused on getting me to move my huge body any way she could. She didn't stand still anymore while I punched the pads, I had to chase her around the ring to do each combination. *Stand still, woman*, I wanted to shout at her. And combinations. We never did them before. This real boxing thing was so hard to remember. Was that left, right, slip, slip, left hook, jab? Or left, right, slip, hook, uppercut, jab? Who knew boxers had to think so much?

And I was having another plateau; I'd had more of them than the Swiss Alps. And my cravings had ramped up. Some people's cravings totally disappear on Banting. Lucky them. I guess I'd messed up my metabolism so much in the past three decades with all my dieting and bingeing that it was going to take a long time to be completely free of cravings, but at least they were now much easier to control and manage than the ones I'd had on all those starvation calorie-reduced diets.

And I had another reason to keep going. My two sisters, who had also struggled with their weight for years, had started seeing Aprille and I felt I had to crack this final hurdle to be a good role model for them. Like me, they had both dieted over the years, often following Oprah's latest fad. Sometimes we even did them together. But of course we always put the weight back on again, just like Oprah.

I adore Oprah. Her passion, her heart, her energy. It was her show that got me to go see my GP about the weird bleeding I was having after giving birth to my daughter. She showed a colonoscopy being done and how it wasn't that awful and then she talked about how awful bowel cancer was, what the symptoms were and how survivable it was if caught early. I was only forty-one and didn't know that bowel cancer ran in my family. I was the first one to get it. I had thought the bleeding was haemorrhoids. A bit more denial going on in my head. I ignored it for six months, and it was seeing that segment on *Oprah* that finally made me go to my doctor.

My GP, Dr Andrew, sent me off for a colonoscopy, which I put off for six weeks. But I did get around to it eventually and when I lay on the table the surgeon introduced himself and asked me about my symptoms. When I told him, a frown flashed across his face before he smiled and said, 'Let's see what's going on for you, then.'

I now know what that frown meant. He knew exactly what he was about to find. My symptom was dark-almost-black blood mixed in with my stool, whereas haemorrhoids are bright red blood. Dark blood is that distinct colour because it has sat in the colon for a while. Luckily the surgeon that day was an amazing bowel cancer expert who took me under his care.

I woke up from the procedure with Russell by my side. 'What are you doing here, darling?' I asked, still groggy from the general anaesthetic. 'Weren't you going to pick me up at the end of your shift?'

'They phoned me at the library and told me to come early,' Russell replied.

We both knew it was bad news. They hadn't asked Russell to come so they could tell us together what a fabulous bowel I had. Mr Stephen, my surgeon, had a pad with a diagram of a bowel on it. He drew a circle and an arrow on the pad to show me where my tumour was. When I go to have my colonoscopy every two years I see that he still has that pad, with a different circle and arrow on it from him having just told someone else they have this very common cancer. Luckily he has never had to use the pad with me again.

After hearing the news Russell and I were in a daze. We couldn't find the way out of the medical centre. We kept walking into storage rooms and toilets for about five minutes before we finally found the exit. It would have been funny in any other circumstance.

We went home and read that bowel cancer has a 50 per cent survival rate once the symptoms appear and an amazing 90 per cent if found pre-symptoms, so everyone should have a regular colonoscopy once they reach forty.

Apart from owing Oprah my life, I also love her because she has struggled with her weight all her life. I've watched her weight go up and down over the years, just like mine. I remember, back in the late eighties, her losing 30 kilos by only drinking liquid protein for four months. I can still picture her taking off that pink jacket and throwing it on the ground as she announced she had reached her goal. The jacket throwing said, *Done! Sorted! Weight problem fixed forever!* She even wheeled a red wagon onto the stage holding 30 kilos of fat to show how much she had lost. She has since admitted she started gorging on food straight after she taped that jacket-throwing episode. Of course she did. She was starving.

By 1992 she was overweight again, having put back on all the weight. She was 107 kilos. She decided exercise was the key and began running half-marathons. So much running. She hired a personal trainer and hit the pavement, but the weight came back again and she then hired a chef who prepared low-fat versions of her favourite foods. I bought the cookbook, of course. She lost weight and so did I, but we both put it back on again. There are only so many days you can get by on a tiny portion of not-fried chicken.

Up and down, up and down her weight went. Then finally she decided that dieting over time makes you fat and that eating sensibly was the key, until she hit menopause and developed a thyroid problem and the sensible eating went out the window.

Most recently she has decided that Weight Watchers is the answer. Weight Watchers! She has bought 10 per cent of the company and sits on the board and does commercials about how this time is going to be different. I watched one of the commercials wondering what it was about Weight Watchers that was now so good. Had they changed what they did? Had they stopped pushing processed foods full of sugar? Nope.

In the commercial Oprah looked and sounded tired. 'If not now, when?' she asked, with a kind of this-is-it-because-it-has-to-be-it desperation.

Oh, Oprah, I wanted to cry at the screen. *Being over fighting your weight does not make a diet work. Wanting it to work with all your might doesn't make it work either.*

'You can eat bread!' she declares in another ad, about the only time she sounds happy. 'I love bread!' Of course she does; she's addicted to it. Drug addicts love crack, it doesn't mean it's good for them.

Oprah, you can't eat bread. My husband can eat bread. Very good quality sourdough bread. But my husband doesn't have a weight problem, plus he hasn't dieted for three decades and therefore become super sensitive to insulin rises and dips. He can eat some bread. *You and I can't, Oprah, not while we are losing weight. We are now too sensitive to carbs, perhaps because we were born that way or because we have made ourselves over-sensitive from swinging between starving ourselves and eating mountains of processed rubbish our whole lives. Once we reach our goal weight then maybe we can have some good quality sourdough every now and then, so long as it doesn't trigger cravings for more.*

Oh, Oprah. With all your money and personal assistants and chefs and trainers and access to the top medical experts – dieting has failed you too, like it fails everyone. I really hope someone tells you about Banting.

We dieters know all about failure. So does the diet industry. Our failure keeps us coming back and paying more. If I started a quit-smoking program in which most of the people who went on it didn't stop smoking and some even ended up smoking more I'd be shut down and I certainly wouldn't be able to advertise on TV and have celebrities endorse my program. How do diet companies keep getting away with making us fatter and making us think the problem is us and not them?

What if we didn't fail all those diets we went on? What if they failed us? What if we didn't have a 'laziness problem', or a 'lack of willpower' problem or a 'lack of exercise' problem? What if we had an 'appetite' problem? What if we had an 'eating the wrong foods that in our bodies cause unmanageable cravings' problem? What if we had a 'hunger hormones' problem? What if we weren't useless and hopeless and lazy, and what if there was a better lifelong solution for our health than the only medical solution – putting a plastic clip on our stomach?

But enough of that and back to me in Melbourne and my plateau. I needed to find a way to break this last plateau so that I could reach my goal of losing at least 40 kilos, be a good role model for my sisters and also so that they didn't get there before me. (I love my sisters very much but there was no way they were going to get to their goal weight before I did.) Aprille said that losing the last bit of weight was the hardest. She said that when I was very overweight and hadn't moved my body for years, even the small changes I made at the start of our work made a big difference. But now, she said, the margins were tighter and I had to work harder to shift the weight.

And she was right. The scale would not budge and my belly was really obvious now that it didn't have those Rock of Gibraltar breasts hiding it. I didn't want to lose much more – I'd lost 37 kilos and just wanted to trim down my belly, which was still a bit large with that bad-for-your-health subcutaneous fat. I'd gone off the idea of a tummy tuck. It felt like cheating. I knew I might revisit the idea when I was down to my final weight, but only if I had a huge amount of loose skin that needed removing.

What to do about this plateau? My eating was perfect. It was second nature now. Aprille said to exercise more often, watch my portion sizes and cut out the snacking. Aprille was becoming a broken record. Or was I just struggling with the same three issues over and over? *Yes*, I realised, *it's me, and not her.*

I decided to cut down on dairy because I suspected I was still quite sensitive to the milk sugars in it and they were driving my cravings. I cut out yoghurt and had two boiled eggs for breakfast instead. That helped. I tried to cut out milk but failed. I couldn't get through the day without at least one dandelion coffee and I couldn't come at having it black.

Then I did a fat fast. This is where you eat only 1200 kilojoules per day and make sure 80 per cent of the food you eat is healthy fat – eggs, fatty cuts of meat, macadamias, salmon, cream cheese and avocado. The other 20 per cent being vegies. I did it for three days and lost 1.5 kilos. You only do a fat fast for three days and only if you are already eating LCHF. It would be too much strain on your gallbladder to do this if you weren't already eating a high level of fat and knew that your body could manage eating a bit more. This is also only recommended to break a plateau. But it has a down side – you are really hungry when it ends and the danger is that you just overeat and put it all back on again, which I pretty much did. And because they have little fibre in them you can also imagine that fat fasts come with another big side effect: constipation.

So, how could I break this final plateau? I needed a goal. A big one. Something to work towards. What about a marathon? I googled marathons and Melbourne. Then I discovered that a marathon is 42.2 kilometres long and remembered that marathon running didn't work for Oprah. I googled fun runs instead. It came up with a few that had just happened and others that were too macho and gave me visions of aggressive runners elbowing the slower runners out of the way. They were fun runs minus the fun and to be avoided. I'd done the 5-kilometre section of the Mother's Day Classic fun run about ten years ago and because I was shuffling so slowly I got caught up in the wave of the

10-kilometre serious runners who all screamed 'Move!' at me as they ran past.

This was my one and only experience of fun runs. Did I really want to do one again? On the Australian Running Calendar website I learned that there was such a thing as women-only runs. I liked the sound of that. I remembered doing a boot camp with a mix of men and women, and doing an exercise where we had to run and grab a flag before our workout partner who was running from the opposite side of the field. My partner was a big bloke but we were equally matched in speed. As we ran towards the flag we both saw we were going to reach it at the same time. I imagined we would grab it together, laugh and say it was a draw, but he had other ideas. We grabbed it, he kneed me in the thigh, I fell to the ground and he grabbed the flag off me, jumped in the air and victory-punched the sky. Nice one. The bruise on my leg took a month to go down. I love blokes – I married one, I gave birth to one – but geez they can be competitive.

I clicked 'women only' and Mudderella came up. It was an American event with army-style obstacle courses, but designed by women for women only. It was coming to Melbourne in December at a big winery an hour out of Melbourne. (Though I didn't think wine was going to be part of the race, somehow.) It would be 9 kilometres long and have sixteen different obstacles you had to slide down, crawl under, rope climb over or swim through. It was happening eleven days before I turned fifty. And there was mud. So much mud. But instead of being aghast at the idea of it I felt my heart beat faster.

Was I really turning fifty at the end of the year? When had that happened? Surely I was only about thirty-six? I felt thirty-six. I checked to see if I was devastated by this huge milestone . . . and I wasn't. Life was good. I had come so far and gained so much – a wonderful family, friends, work, my writing, a terrific community and renewed health and fitness. I was very lucky. Fifty was actually a badge of honour. A great achievement.

I signed up and emailed my friend Caroline to ask if she wanted to roll around in the mud with me for 11 kilometres. Surprisingly, she did.

Did anyone else want to? I registered a team then told other friends I was doing this to celebrate losing so much weight and to do something crazy before I turned fifty. Our friend Alex was in too. No one else was crazy enough to join us.

How do you train for an event like that? You run. And run. And run. And that's what I did.

And how did we go at Mudderella? There was mud. So much mud. Up to our armpits in mud. Crawling on our knees in mud. Literally swimming in deep, deep mud. We slipped, we slid, we fell face first. But we got up. Over and over. A bit like life, really. A bit like losing weight.

We got dirtier than we have ever wanted to get, ever. It took three showers to get it all off. We also laughed a lot. We didn't get hurt, apart from me swallowing a fly right at the start. No one screamed at us to move out of the way. No one timed us or treated it like a race to the finish. Other teams helped us and we helped them and each other. And that's why we finished. Not first. Not last. But we did it.

How many more metaphors can I make comparing a mud-based obstacle course to losing weight?

Just one.

Mudderella's theme is Find Your Strong.

I found mine. And boy is it strong.

Chapter Twelve

82 kilos

So, I made it. Here I am at my final weight. Not a Size 0 super-model, but slim and healthy having lost 40 kilos. This was never about vanity but rather about living to see my kids grow up and being able to grow old with my husband – surely the best part of finding your soulmate.

Playing soccer with my son at the park one night, I felt so light and free. 'I'm playing soccer!' I shouted as I dodged and weaved to chase the ball.

'Stop embarrassing me,' my son hissed back as he took the ball off me, but I couldn't help it. It was so wonderful to be a normal size it made me feel like shouting from the rooftops. And it still does.

'I'm walking easily through the train barriers!'

'I'm buying size 14 jeans!'

'I'm shopping at the front of the bra shop!'

I can't tell you how good it is to feel normal, to not be

embarrassed when I meet new people, or bump into old friends I haven't seen for ages.

When I was at my heaviest and I'd pass an obese woman on the street I used to discreetly ask Russell, 'Am I as big as her?' Russell, God bless him, would always say no. But when he paused before he answered, I knew he was lying. Asking these questions was all part of my denial: *At least I'm not as bad as that poor woman.*

I don't play this game anymore. I'm no longer free-falling towards death and finding fleeting relief by pointing out someone who is going to beat me to it.

It's little moments every day that tell me how far I have come, such as being able to wrap a normal-sized towel around myself as I dash from the bathroom to my bedroom hoping none of the neighbours can see – sorry, neighbours, I will try to remember to pull the curtains!

It's being able to run around the park after my kids. It's being able to buy nice bathers, not the horrible swirly shockers at the back of the shop. It's being able to sit in a chair and not worry about how I will get out of it.

But the best thing is being mostly free from food cravings. Not thinking about food every waking hour frees up so much time and energy. And feeling calm and in control around food is priceless.

I feel so blessed to have found Aprille and so grateful that her approach was Banting. If she had made me weigh food and eat sugar-filled low-fat yoghurts I probably would have lasted a few weeks then ditched her and the whole idea of ever being at a healthy weight.

I now eat mindfully, always thinking about what I am putting in my mouth. Not in an obsessive way, but in a calm, clear way, just asking myself the gentle question, 'Is this the best thing I can put in my body right now?' On all the diets I've gone on I always looked forward to reaching my goal weight when I could stop thinking about my food choices, which was probably one of the reasons I always put weight straight back on again after losing it. I always saw making food choices as a chore, a punishment, a supreme restriction. Now it is second nature.

When I reflect back on all those diets I can't believe the rubbish foods they had me eating. Pre-packaged, mass-produced foods that are full of sugar. Plus, having so many items that mimic cheap takeaways and treats – such as pizza, pasta, fish and chips, sausage rolls, ice-cream, biscuits and chocolate bars – is about sucking the overweight into thinking they don't have to change the way they eat to lose weight. Something I fell for again and again. You *do* have to change the way you eat. Eating low-fat versions of rubbish foods is no way to lose weight and keep it off.

I am also grateful that I found Mischa's gym, a place where I felt supported and never judged. I know not everyone can afford a personal trainer and a nutritionist, and I was very lucky to have that double support. But exercise can be as simple as walking around the block or swimming at the local pool, all activities that helped me on my journey. Diet may be 80 per cent of losing weight, but exercise still plays a vital role as well as having many health benefits and making you feel strong and powerful, which will help you stick to your goals. Moving my body helped me own it, which was crucial to taking control of my health.

And I'm so grateful to Russell, for his love and support and amazing cooking. Not everyone has a Russell in the kitchen cooking beautiful meals for them. I wish I could clone him for you, but I can't. And even if I could, you can't have him – he's mine.

I am also grateful to my car park epiphany. But to be honest, I had hundreds of epiphanies: when I couldn't climb the stairs at work, when clothing didn't fit, when someone I hadn't seen for ages stared at me horrified when we bumped into each other in a local park. I'm glad the car park epiphany finally made me commit to action.

The absolute best thing about this journey is no longer having that voice in my head that tells me to eat all the time. That voice was so hard to ignore, but giving in to it never made it go away, in fact it made it worse.

If I had one piece of advice for anyone wanting to lose weight, it would be to find the small forgotten voice even deeper down inside, smothered by years of failure and self-criticism, drowned out by the too-easy promises of the weight-loss industry – the voice that says you deserve a healthy body and a happy relationship with food. That food is wonderful and nourishing and an essential part of life. Listen to that voice. And keep listening to it. That is your true self speaking.

Part Two

How you can free yourself from your prison of fat

If you're anything like me you've read Part 1 thinking, *When will she get to the bit about how to lose weight? Get to the damn diet!*

But this isn't a diet.

What?! I paid good money for this book and it isn't a diet! (This is you again, just to be clear.)

No, it isn't a diet. (Me now.) A diet is something you do short term, for a few weeks, a few months or maybe even for a whole miserable year. You starve. You weigh every morsel you put in your mouth. You constantly try to work out different ways to put your food on the scale so it weighs less and you can eat more. You know what I mean – if I pile the boiled chicken pieces in the middle of the scale does it weigh more than if I put it in four equal piles in the corners of the scale?

And you manage to starve for a while and you lose weight and you are irritable and tired and oh-so-hungry all the time. And maybe you reach your goal weight or maybe you fall short and then you start eating everything in sight and you can't stop. You literally can't stop.

And the weight comes back much faster than you lost it. And you are ashamed and so cross with yourself, but still you can't stop eating. And people no longer ask how the diet is going because it obviously isn't going anymore and of course you told everyone you were on a diet because this was going to be the time you finally lost weight for good.

So, now you have public shame to match your private shame. But actually, deep down, all through the starving and the food weighing, you knew this diet would fail. They all fail. A diet is a short-term fix that isn't a fix at all because it will always end in failure. It always has and it always will. Because any kind of calorie-reduced eating sends your body even further into starvation mode and it fights back with its huge arsenal of hunger hormones, and those hormones play dirty.

My nutritionist Aprille said to me in our first session, 'This isn't a diet. This is a way of life.'

She's right.

This is about taking control, healing your body, working with your hormones, not against them, and stopping the constant battle with yourself, your body, your food and your self-esteem. This is about freedom. This is about being a healthy weight and saying goodbye to cravings.

To understand why Banting works you first need to understand the science behind it, so I have devoted a whole chapter to this. I know you will want to skip to the 'What do I eat?' section but please don't. It is vitally important for you to understand why it is really bad to eat that one cupcake and why it is okay if you are tired/stressed/hungry/bored to grab a handful of nuts or a chunk of cheese or an avocado.

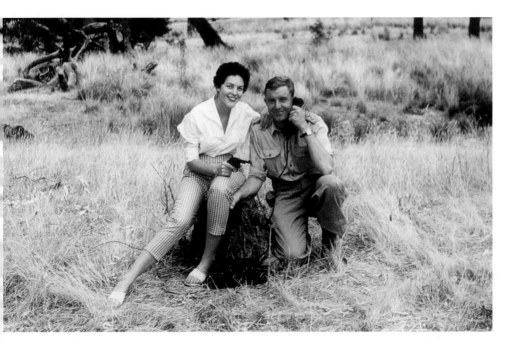

My parents, Mary and Michael, in 1961 just after their engagement. Mum's brother John had driven her up to the army training camp at Puckapunyal, central Victoria, to see Dad. John joked that Mum should hold Dad up with his army gun so he couldn't get out of the engagement.

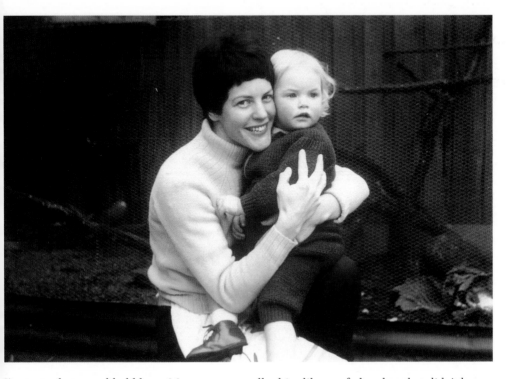

I'm around a year old old here. Mum was naturally thin, like my father, but that didn't last for either of them sadly.

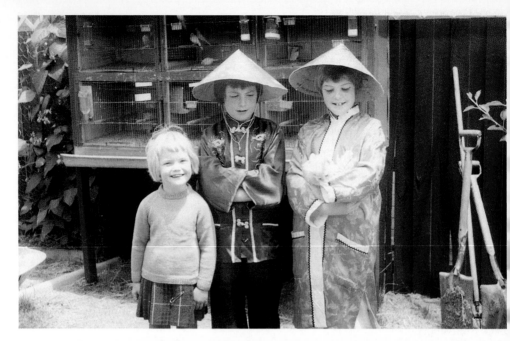

This was taken in 1970 in our backyard when I was four. My two sisters, Helen (centre) and Ruth (right) were going to a dress-up party. I was upset that I wasn't going until Mum put a bit of red cloth on my head and told me I was now dressed up too. I was thrilled! Ruth is holding our new cat, Smoky. We are all a healthy weight.

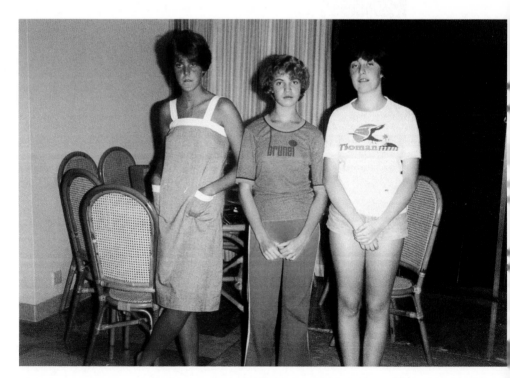

Three teenage sisters not too happy about Dad taking our photo. By now I was 12 (centre) and we were living in Singapore. All very trim.

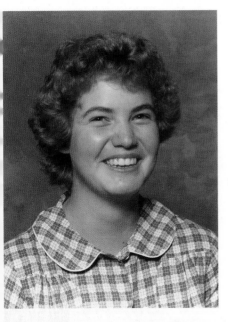

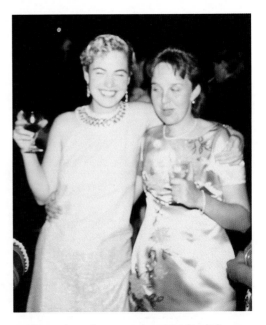

Back from Singapore at the age of 14.
Putting on weight for the first time and
hating myself for it.

With my friend Katie at her 21st birthday
party. I'm 20 and at my skinniest, thinking
my teenage puppy fat phase is over forever.

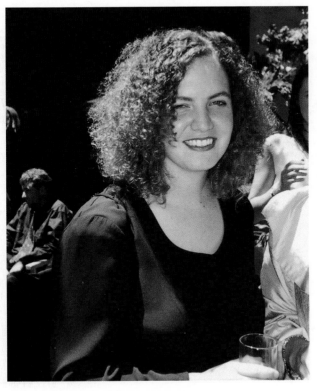

Me at the age of 30 at my cousin Meredith's wedding.
The puppy fat is back and here to stay.

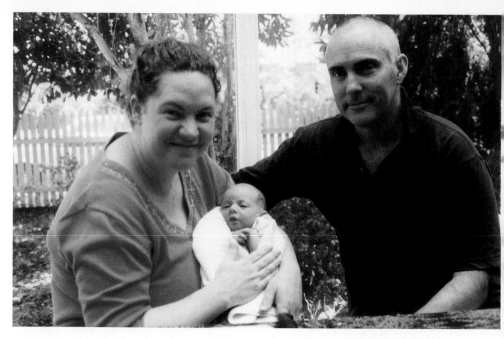

Russell and me in 2002 just after our son was born. The baby weight has started to pile on.

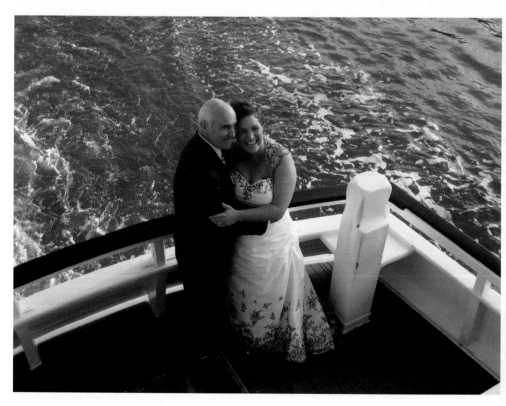

Our wedding day in 2008. Such a lovely day but I'd just had my second child and still couldn't shift that baby weight, even for such a special occasion.

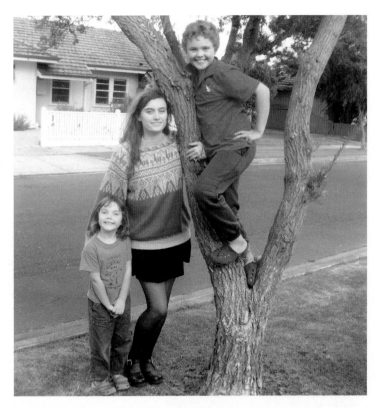

My two gorgeous children with their equally gorgeous half-sister.

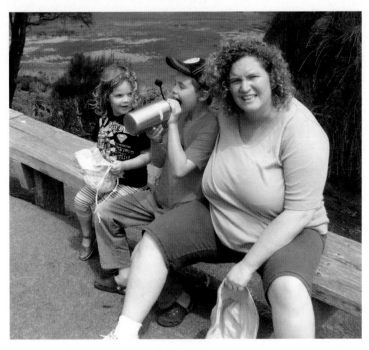

On a family holiday in 2012. We had just climbed Tower Hill near Warnambool. It's only 80 metres high but I was completely puffed!

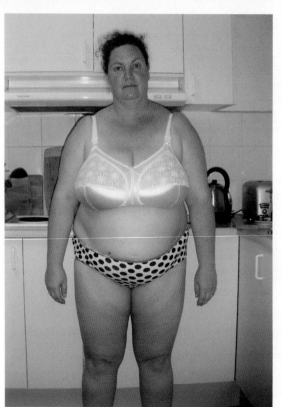

The fridge photo – front view! I got Russell to take this when I was at my heaviest and put it on the fridge as a reminder to lose weight. It stayed there for a whole day until a friend came over and I whipped it off.

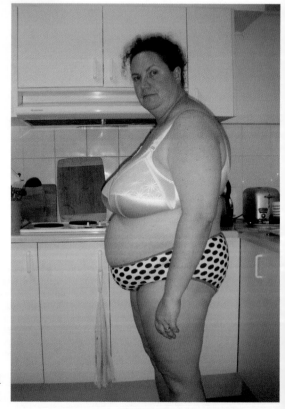

The fridge photo – side view. Check out that stomach . . . and those spotty undies!

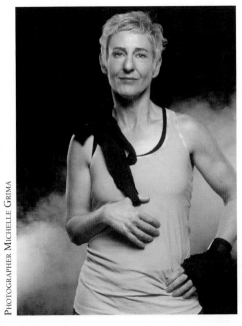

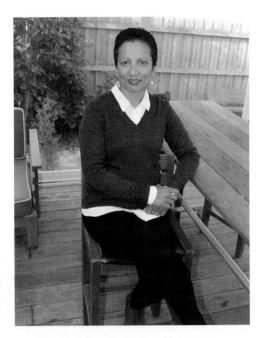

PHOTOGRAPHER MICHELLE GRIMA

But then I met this lady (top left): Mischa Merz, ex-champion boxer and awesome personal trainer. And this lady (top right): Aprille McMahon, radical nutritionist and life-changer.

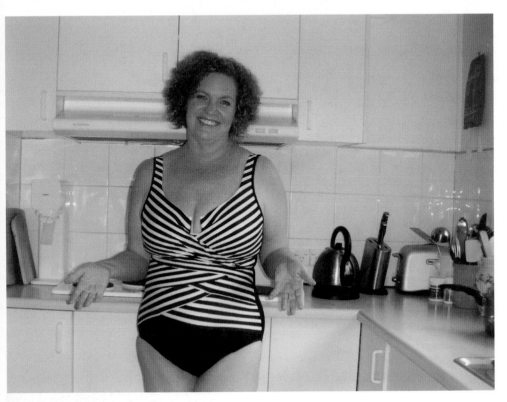

And here's my fridge shot again, 36 kilos lighter.

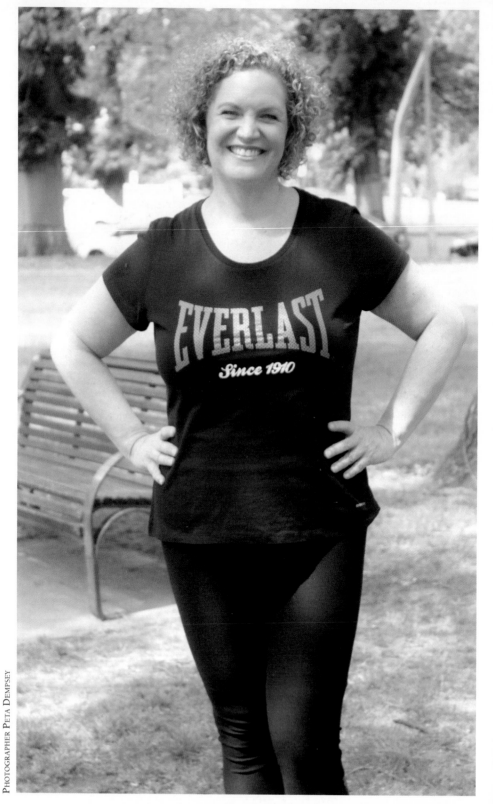

PHOTOGRAPHER PETA DEMPSEY

Here I am again in my running gear, having lost 40 kilos. So many reasons to smile!

Read the science, then follow my tips and Aprille's recipes and meal plans.

I know you've read lots of weight-loss books that have promised they had THE ANSWER and they didn't. But this next section does; it is the key to your gaol cell. I can't say this enough: YOU WILL NEVER DIET AGAIN. You will learn to love food and not resent it. This is freedom.

After the science you'll find food lists of what you can eat, what foods you need to ditch and some great new foods you can embrace. And I actually mean embrace. I have discovered the most delicious butter chicken in the world; Russell once sprung me hugging a bowl of it. I wish that was a joke. During my weight-loss journey I have also been known to hug other foods, especially a big bowl of konjac noodles (see page 227) smothered in carbonara sauce and cheese – one of my new comfort foods.

The fantastic thing is that now my comfort foods actually love me back.

Chapter Thirteen

The Science of Banting/LCHF

Insulin is a fat-storing hormone. Let me say that again, in capitals this time. INSULIN IS A FAT-STORING HORMONE. Previously it has been your worst enemy. It has been Ghengis Khan and you've been a poor villager dressed in rags, clutching a stick, hiding in your straw hut and hoping the sound of thundering hooves coming over the mountain pass was just in your imagination.

Insulin, or too much of it to be precise, is one reason you are fat and yet you constantly crave food. Yes, of course genetics, stress, environment, inactivity, lack of quality sleep, gut bacteria, certain medications and some medical conditions like polycystic ovarian syndrome or an underactive thyroid will contribute to your weight and hunger. You can't change some factors in your life but you can absolutely influence how much insulin your body pumps out.

I am going to go on and on about insulin. I'm going to explain how you have been riding an insulin fat-storing rollercoaster that goes up and down but mostly up. And I'm going to tell you how you can get off it for good and get your insulin under control.

Insulin 101

Insulin is a hormone that is made in the pancreas. If you have the same denial relationship with your body that I had, you probably won't know what or where your pancreas is. It's in your abdomen – that's the big bulging thing you suck in every time you have your photo taken. It sits behind your stomach. It's close to the stomach for a very good reason because its main role is to help your body digest food, particularly protein. It also makes and releases insulin.

I am going to take a little sidestep here and quickly talk about protein and the other two big components of food – fat and carbo-hydrates. If you've been on every diet known to man you probably know the fat/protein/carb composition of every food on the planet but, again, bear with me, this is important stuff.

Foods are comprised of the following nutrients: fats, protein, carbohydrates, water, minerals and vitamins. The first three are the macronutrients, the things your body needs in large quanti-ties; vitamins and minerals are the micronutrients, the things you need in small quantities. These three macronutrients – fat, protein and carbs – provide energy. Every cell in your body, including your muscles and tissues, needs energy. How much energy a food has is measured in kilojoules or calories, depending on whether you use the metric or the imperial system.

Before we get back to the pancreas (yes, I know you are dying to learn more about it), let's take a closer look at those three compo-nents that make up 90 per cent of the food we eat.

Carbohydrates, which your body converts into glucose (sugar).

Protein, which your body converts into amino acids (the building blocks of our cells that are essential to healing, building muscle and organ function).

Fat, which your body converts into fatty acids (an essential energy source that is also used to rebuild and create new cells).

The weight-loss industry has taught you that you just need to reduce your kilojoule/calorie intake to lose weight. And that the composition of the food doesn't actually matter so long as the calories are low. So, a 22-gram Weight Watchers Cherry and Dark Choc Delight Cherry Flavoured Indulgent Bar (yes, that really is its name) with its 90 calories is much better for weight loss than eating 22 grams of macadamia nuts that has 158 calories. Remember those two foods. Once you know everything there is to know about insulin and your pancreas we are going to follow those two foods through your digestive system and see exactly what they do to your body, remembering that the weight-loss industry tells you that the cherry-flavoured bar is good for weight loss and the macadamias are bad.

The bar is a food high in processed carbs, and before we get back to the pancreas I just want to outline the difference between a processed carb and an unprocessed carb. Processed carb foods are foods that either: 1. Come in a package and have a list of ingredients on the side. 2. Last a long time if you leave them on the bench. 3. Have a long shelf life and are kept in the pantry rather than the fridge. There are a few exceptions to this. Eggs (which are very low in carbs), for example, are great for you and don't necessarily have to be kept in the fridge. Unprocessed food – real food that contains carbs, such as eggs, nuts, seeds, vegetables and fruit – still looks like it is supposed to look. A machine hasn't created them. Dairy also falls into the real-food category even though there is a fair amount of processing that goes into producing dairy products; this is because their nutritional value is important to us.

Now, back to the pancreas.

It's shaped a bit like an apostrophe lying on its side, fat at one end with a long body and a curly tail. It's about 25 centimetres long.

The pancreas has two jobs. Once food has been partially digested by the stomach, it is pushed into the small intestine. The pancreas then adds its own digestive juices and enzymes to the food. That's the pancreas's first job. Good on you, pancreas, but we are not interested in that. We are interested in its second job – producing the hormone insulin, which helps to control the amount of glucose (sugar) in the blood.

Excess glucose that remains in the blood is toxic. The body needs to deal with it and deal with it quickly. Even if you think about eating food full of easily digestible glucose your pancreas starts sending out insulin. When you take your first bite of a carbohydrate it sends out more, and even more if it is a processed carb. When the carb-filled food begins to break down in the stomach and enters the top of the small intestine where its sugar finally hits your bloodstream the pancreas shoots out even more insulin. Insulin signals all cells in your body that there is rapid energy available and to open up and take it in. When you eat or drink something that is broken down quickly to glucose, a flood of insulin is needed so that the now high blood glucose can be brought back to normal quickly. But it also does something else. Something that is making you fat. This is the most important piece of information in this whole chapter. Insulin release stimulates the storage of fatty acids in the form of triglycerides – this is the main way your body stores fat.

That makes total sense and should work really well and does in lean people. Once the body uses up the glucose, the pancreas stops releasing insulin. This absence of glucose tells the fat stores that the crisis is over and they can go back to doing their job of releasing steady amounts of fatty acids for energy. Previously you've been taught to think of the fat storage areas of your body as some sort of rainy-day famine larder where the body puts excess energy in case tomorrow or next week or next year it finds itself starving. This is questionable. Energy, as fatty acids, goes in and out of your fat cells all the time. Or it should. What helps fat to be used as energy is the absence of glucose in the blood. This is what we want. We want no glucose around so that your body's energy needs can come more from the excess fat you have stored.

And this is where those of us with weight and hunger problems fall in a heap. High levels of insulin over time are problematic. Cells stop responding to insulin, particularly when surrounded by excess fat. Messenger-receiving molecules in the fat-covered cells don't work as well, so the glucose doesn't get taken up. This is a feature of type-2 diabetes. This means that the pancreas makes more insulin because it still wants to get rid of the glucose that is hanging around in the blood, so it instructs the liver to turn the glucose into triglycerides and sends it to fat storage.

And through all this the cells in your body haven't got the energy they need. So, you eat some more processed carbs, your blood sugar goes up, your insulin goes up pretty quickly and you feel great because you've got energy at your disposal again and because glucose stimulates 'feel good' mood chemicals in your brain called dopamine and serotonin. Not surprisingly, glucose then goes down pretty quickly too and you feel hungry again. But you haven't 'fed' your cells properly, you've just stored some fat and your cells are still looking for energy, so you look for processed carbs again to curb the hunger. Your blood glucose goes up, insulin goes up, fat storage happens, glucose crashes, cells are hungry, you feel hungry and you eat processed carbs again . . . See the pattern?

And one food type spikes insulin more than anything else – highly processed readily digested carbohydrates.

And the answer?

Stop eating them. Stop building up your fat stores and let your fat stores send good stable fatty acid energy to all the cells in your body.

This is where a conservative nutritionist would say, *Just don't eat sugary processed carbs and you will be fine. You can still eat wholegrain carbs in plentiful amounts.* But our systems are so out of whack and we are so sensitive to carbs that for many people this isn't a solution. Complex carbohydrates will still spike your insulin, just not as quickly. Proteins spike it too, but more slowly, and fructose – the sugar in fruit and other foods – goes straight to the liver to be turned into fat and stored there, and any excess that the liver can't handle gets deposited around other organs and tissues.

The food that helps to keep our insulin under control is fat.

Beautiful, comfort-giving, makes-you-feel-full fat.

That is a lot to take in, so let's look at it step by step.

What happens when you eat if you have a happy, balanced, lean body:

1. You eat.
2. Your pancreas secretes insulin.
3. The insulin signals the cells to open up and take in energy as glucose from the bloodstream.
4. The insulin also signals the fat cells to stop releasing energy as fatty acids into the bloodstream.
5. Any glucose not used up gets turned into fatty acids and sent to the fatty stores for use at a later time.
6. The levels of glucose in the bloodstream drop and the pancreas stops producing insulin.

7. No insulin around signals the fat stores to release fatty acids again for the cells to use as fuel until you eat again.

Now let's look at what happens in a body that is out of whack, comes from a gene pool of people who easily get fat and has been subjected to heavy loads of quick-energy processed carbs over many years:

1. You eat.
2. Your pancreas secretes insulin.
3. The insulin signals the cells to open up and take in energy as glucose from the bloodstream.
4. The cells don't pay attention because they have become insulin resistant, and insulin stays high.
5. Your cells are now screaming for energy because the fat surrounding those cells is not allowing the glucose to get in.
6. The pancreas recognises that the blood-sugar levels are still high and releases even more insulin to tell the body it is an emergency. The body responds by converting the glucose to triglycerides and storing it as fat.
7. Your brain releases hunger hormones and you have cravings for high-energy quick-releasing glucose foods.
8. You eat high-energy quick-releasing glucose foods.
9. It all starts over again and goes on and on and on . . .

Through all this eating your cells are constantly starving. This is called insulin resistance and many people who are obese have this condition. Anything that keeps insulin levels high in this cycle of cravings will actually increase your ability to store fat and decrease your ability to burn fat.

How do we reverse this? How do we stop all this insulin telling the fat stores to hold their fat, sending glucose to the liver, depriving your body of energy and creating even more fat stores to hold even more fat? We do everything we can to try to stop the body from releasing these huge amounts of insulin.

We eliminate processed carbohydrates, instead getting carbs mostly from nuts, seeds, eggs, dairy, vegetables and some fruit. We eat moderate amounts of protein, because excess protein spikes insulin. And we eat good fats, which have the least effect on insulin and fill us up, make us feel full and provide steady energy to the body and brain.

But won't eating fat make me fat? Won't it go straight to my fat cells? Not necessarily. Fat is converted into fatty acids for the body to use immediately as energy or sent to your fat stores for use later on in the day. And remember that there is no insulin telling those fat stores to close up, so your body can access those fatty acids when it needs them.

And here's something Weight Watchers won't tell you: you can eliminate processed carbs because everything you eat except animal flesh has a carbohydrate value. This means that when you eat, you are always getting carbs but just the good ones – the unprocessed ones. So, until now you have been eating processed carbs that make you hungry and overweight and it's something you don't need!

You don't need processed carbohydrates. Let's put that in capitals too: YOU DON'T NEED PROCESSED CARBOHYDRATES.

Some nutritionists will say you should eat all food groups, including processed carbohydrates such as bread, in moderation. This needs some clarification. In a balanced diet you need a generous amount of good fats, a moderate amount of protein and a smaller amount of unprocessed carbs. Cutting out processed carbs works like fat-burning magic, except it isn't magic, it is something that was known for hundreds of years before the grain industry got involved with making the American food pyramid in 1977. The result was that we were all taught that eating three to five servings of vegetables per day (pretty low), two to four servings of fruit (pretty high) and six to eleven servings of grains (insanely high) was 'essential' to our health.

Let's go back to those macadamia nuts now, along with that choc-cherry-flavoured bar. The bar has thirty different ingredients. Thirty! The macadamias have one ingredient and that would be, just let me look on the packet . . . oh, that's right, there is no packet . . . it has macadamia nut in it. Those 22 grams of nuts are made up of 17 grams of fat, 1 gram of net carbohydrates and 2 grams of protein. When you eat it you get a minor release of insulin and your body can keep using fat as its energy source. The result is an absence of glucose, an absence of insulin and a body that is less likely to store fat. Your fat stores don't stop releasing fatty acids and your cells don't stop getting energy from the freely circulating fatty acids. And your fat stores get more fuel to release when the body needs it throughout the coming day and night.

The thirty ingredients in the Weight Watchers Cherry and Dark Choc Delight Cherry Flavoured Indulgent Bar:

sugar, vegetable oil, cocoa powder, milk solids, emulsifier 492, soy lecithin, natural flavour, concentrated apple puree, cherry puree, concentrated elderberry juice, sorbitol (a **sugar** alcohol from fruit), glycerol (liquid sugar, used as an emollient and laxative, and for making explosives and antifreeze), invert **sugar** (a sweeter tasting **sugar**), polydextrose (a type of **sugar**), sunflower oil, wheat fibre, pectin, calcium lactate, citric acid, rolled oats, rice, salt, malt barley extract (another type of **sugar**), maltodextrin (can be classed as **sugar** depending on how it is made), coconut, preservative 223, dextrose (concentrated **sugar**), emulsifier 471, blackcurrant juice concentrate, honey (**sugar**)

That's eight different types of sugar in one 22-gram bar!

Now let's follow that choc-cherry-flavoured bar down into your stomach. It contains 1 gram of protein, 3 grams of fat and a whopping 13 grams of carbs. That's over 3 teaspoons of sugar. (One teaspoon is 4 grams.) That's an all-out insulin party right there. Blood sugar goes up, insulin goes up, fat use goes down, fat storage goes up and very soon you want more. You get ravenous and think about having another one. Hey, they're only 2 pro points, after all, maybe you could skip lunch and have two? Or maybe you could have three and skip dinner as well? See what's happening here?

On the cherry-bar pack, under the title 'Handy Hints', Weight Watchers gives the following advice:

- Keep a bar on standby at work or at home.
- Perfect for morning AND afternoon coffee breaks.
- Sweet treat after meals.

The capitals above are mine not theirs, but you get the idea. Weight Watchers isn't even pretending this is a once-in-a-blue-moon snack. They are suggesting you have this thirty-ingredient 13-grams-of-carbs mess every day!

It also says on the pack, 'Life is too short to pass on the treats.' Your life will be short if you *don't* pass on this kind of treat. This is where you might be thinking that you can eat all day long so long as you don't spike your insulin. Sorry, that isn't the case. Fat and protein still contain energy and it has to go somewhere, and if you don't need it today that energy will remain in your fat stores as fat.

So, you do need to watch the amount of food you eat on Banting/LCHF, but here's the good bit. If you keep your insulin under control, your body won't be screaming for energy, turning on the hunger hormones and making you eat lots of bad foods.

The secret to LCHF is that it reduces your hunger and you eat less.

That's the magic. Right there.

You don't think about food all day long. You don't constantly make deals with yourself like, *If I have that one chocolate biscuit I promise to go for a run after work*, and then you eat five biscuits and are too sluggish to run because of the dramatic fluctuations in your blood-sugar levels.

Here's the not-so-good bit. If you want to reduce the fat stores your body has built up, you have to eat less than your body needs, to encourage it to dip into those stores and reduce them. But remember, those stores are now open for business and you only have to eat a little less each day until you get lean. And you will get lean, trust me.

Then, once at your goal weight, you eat exactly what your body needs each day and no more. And your body will communicate this to you calmly and quietly, not screaming at you 24/7 that it is starving.

I just want to say one last thing, and it's about the C word. No, not *that* C word! Cholesterol. People will say that if you are eating saturated fat then surely your arteries will clog and you will die of a heart attack. That's the biggest criticism levelled at this kind of eating, but it isn't necessarily correct. Rumours were even spread around the world when Dr Robert Atkins died that it was because of a heart attack. His way of eating is much higher protein than Banting/LCHF but he didn't die of a heart attack. He died at the age of seventy-two from a fall, hitting his head on an icy New York pavement.

Cholesterol is found at the site of damaged artery walls but that doesn't mean it caused the damage. That's like saying fire fighters are the ones who light fires because they are always seen at the site of them. Inflammation is what causes artery walls to become inflamed. Easily digested high-energy processed carbohydrates, such as sugar and packaged foods, and the insulin they bring into your blood, are incredibly inflammatory. Another food that is very inflammatory is trans-fats, which Banting/LCHF excludes completely. Trans-fats do occur naturally in very small amounts in animal products but are mass created in an industrial process that adds hydrogen to liquid vegetable oils to make them more solid. The artificial kind is used heavily in processed foods and commercially to deep fry food as the oil can be used over and over.

Cholesterol is in fact a type of fat that is part of all animal cells. It is essential for many of the body's metabolic processes, including the making of hormones, bile and vitamin D. Cholesterol can't dissolve in the blood. It must be transported through your blood by carriers called lipoproteins. The two main types of lipoproteins that carry cholesterol to and from cells are low-density lipoproteins (LDL), and high-density lipoproteins (HDL). LDL is often called the bad cholesterol and HDL the good cholesterol. This way of eating may increase your good (HDL) cholesterol and may even increase your overall cholesterol but it is your triglyceride-to-HDL ratio that is a better indicator of your risk of heart disease. You need to keep this below 2.5, and this way of eating brings that ratio down in most people.

A small subset of people who eat LCHF do experience increased levels of bad (LDL) cholesterol. Hence the importance of regular cholesterol checks. That way you smile confidently when people tell you mistakenly that you will have a heart attack by eating this way, and can also ensure you are not in that small subset whose cholesterol is negatively affected by this way of eating.

Right. That's the science done. Phew. Thanks for bearing with me.

Chapter Fourteen

How having an overweight or obese body could be killing you

Not being in denial about your body is such an important step towards taking control of your health. You may want to sing *la la la* loudly and stick your fingers in your ears instead of reading this chapter, but please don't. Being overweight or obese is very bad for your health. Do I have a new study that has just proved it? You know I do!

It is called 'The Duration of Adult Overweight, Obesity and Cancer Risk in the Women's Health Initiative: A Longitudinal Study from the United States'. This study investigated the cancer risk of the overweight and obese participants in The Women's Health Initiative (WHI). The WHI was a major fifteen-year research program that looked at the most common causes of death, disability and poor quality of life in 161,808 generally healthy postmenopausal women.

What it found was shocking. For every decade a woman is obese, her odds of developing breast, endometrial, colon or kidney cancer rises by 10 per cent. For each decade she's overweight, her risk rises by 7 per cent. Those are both huge increases in risk.

This study is not alone in this finding. Many other studies have shown that being overweight or obese is second only to smoking as a danger to your health and to developing cancer and heart disease.

And unfortunately the news gets even worse. Many overweight and obese people have other risk factors, such as being inactive and eating a poor diet that even further increases their chances of developing ill health.

So, why is being overweight or obese so bad for you?

Obesity is bad for your body on several different fronts. Some cancers, especially breast, endometrial and uterine cancers, are sensitive to the female sex hormone estrogen. The National Institute of Environmental Health Sciences (NIEHS) in America actually added estrogen to its list of known cancer-causing agents in 2002. This natural hormone, that half the world produces, isn't always carcinogenic; this occurs only in certain circumstances, and guess what? Fat cells produce an excess of estrogen.

But it doesn't stop there. Fat cells were once thought to be benign, that all they did was hang around storing excess energy. This is not so. Fat tissue is metabolically active, secreting hormones and inflammatory cytokines. These hormones and cytokines affect various parts of the body resulting in inflammation, which can contribute to cancer growth and heart disease. Eating LCHF is very good for reducing inflammation.

There's more. Obese and overweight people love sugar, and so, it seems, does cancer. Sugar may be its favourite food for fuel. Some experts believe that eating a high-sugar diet could encourage cancer growth whereas avoiding sugar may starve it. The 1931

Nobel Laureate in Medicine was awarded to Dr Otto Warburg, who discovered that cancer cells have a very different energy metabolism compared to healthy cells. He found that malignant tumors have increased glycolysis, a process whereby glucose is used as a fuel. PET (positron emission tomography) scans are one of the most accurate tools for detecting cancer growth. In a PET scan a patient drinks a radioactive-laced glucose drink to detect sugar-hungry tumor cells in their body.

Plus, people with weight problems tend to snack or graze all day long and therefore don't give their body the essential time it needs to heal and repair damaged cells. Research has shown that cycles of prolonged fasting protect against immune-system damage and induce immune-system regeneration. A study from the University of Southern California concluded that fasting shifts stem cells from a dormant state to a state of self-renewal. This study was conducted on chemotherapy patients and involved prolonged periods of not eating, but it does show how the body regenerates when not digesting food. I never eat after 8pm and eat breakfast at 8am. A twelve-hour fast every day. When I was obese I was still shovelling in food at ten o'clock at night and going to sleep on a full stomach.

These are all good reasons to reduce your waistline and your eating, get your insulin levels down and work on any other risk factors you might have – by exercising regularly, eating wholesome real foods and not smoking.

You may say that it isn't guaranteed that being overweight or obese will make you sick; that it is only a risk. But is it a risk worth taking? If you are thinking of giving up on LCHF, come back and read this chapter again. It's not long. It will only take you a few minutes and might save your life.

We should all live long, happy lives, and your chances of doing that are so much greater if you are not overweight or obese.

153

Chapter Fifteen

Foods to embrace, foods to have occasionally and foods to run screaming from

The main thing to remember is to eat real foods. Real foods don't come in a packet and they don't have thirty different ingredients that you need a science degree to be able to understand.

There's a great saying that you shouldn't eat anything your grandmother wouldn't recognise. Okay, neither of my grandmothers would have recognised konjac noodles (see page 227), but that's only because they weren't Japanese.

The foods to embrace

Here's the best bit. Food to love that will love you back.

Meat
All meat and game, all parts of the animal including the skin and

the fat. Cured meats such as bacon, sausage (but check what's in it in case it has rice flour or some other starch), chorizo, pancetta and parma ham are also good too, though Aprille suggests limiting bacon to twice per week. The only exceptions are highly processed meats, often cured with a lot of sugar and full of fillers and preservatives, such as luncheon meats. Don't eat them. Do buy the best quality meat you can afford, preferably grass-fed and organic.

Fish and shellfish

Pass the prawns, please! And the scallops, mussels, oysters, clams, shrimps, crayfish and lobster. All fish are great, preferably wild-caught, but fatty fish such as salmon are particularly good. Eat them any way you like, just don't coat them with flour and bread-crumbs. Watch out for tinned fish in an olive-oil blend; the word 'blend' refers to soy oil. Tuna in pure olive oil is hard to find but worth the search.

Eggs

The humble egg. Nature's perfect food. It keeps for weeks and can be poached, fried, steamed or baked. A 63-gram egg contains 6 grams of fat, 8 grams of protein, 0 grams of carbs, every vitamin except vitamin C, plus selenium, folate, biotin, calcium, cephalin, iodine, sodium, phosphorous, iron, thiamine and zinc. One of the few things it doesn't have is fibre, and a side serve of spinach can fix that. A good day starts with eggs. We get ours from our four chickens: Doctor Speckles, Big Red, Snow White and Honey Chicken. We no longer have Crispy Chicken. *She* turned out to be a *he* and started crowing at 5am each morning and didn't stop until sunset. Crispy is now living on a farm and lording it over our friend Beau's flock of hens. There is nothing like an egg straight from the nest, poached with a touch of vinegar and served on a bed of fried mushrooms. If you don't have Doctor Speckles and friends giving you fresh eggs daily, don't despair, get good quality free-range eggs from the supermarket, health-food shop or farmers market. Learn to love eggs. They are nature's little present to you.

Natural fats to eat and cook with

This is the good bit. The oh-my-goodness-I-thought-these-things-were-really-bad-for-me-but-now-I can-eat-them bit. Butter, cream, coconut oil, olive oil, avocado oil, macadamia oil, lard, ghee, duck fat or any rendered animal fat. (There are two ways to render fat you get from the butcher or a farmer: the wet method or the dry method. Google 'how to render fat' for the different methods.) Once you eat food prepared with these good fats you will wonder how you ever ate stuff from a packet full of cheap trans-fats.

Vegetables that grow above ground

The rule of thumb here is: if it grows above ground, love it; if it grows below ground be wary of it. But like all thumbs (and fingers) this rule can be broken (see the sometimes food list below). The excellent chow-down vegies are the green leafies: spinach, kale, all the lettuces and Swiss Chard (no, I don't know what that is either); and the cruciferous vegies: cauliflower, cabbage, bok choy, broccoli, Brussels sprouts. These others are equally awesome: asparagus, zucchini, celery, eggplant, olives (yes, technically a fruit but still good), mushrooms, cucumber, avocado and capsicum. Avocados are especially good with their 29 grams of fat and only 4 grams of protein and 4 grams of net carbs.

Dairy

I'm talking about the real thing, not rubbish processed dairy-like creations such as ice-cream or frozen yoghurt. Full fat and close to nature, so milk, butter, cream, sour cream, double cream, Greek yogurt and high-fat cheeses such as camembert, feta, cheddar, Jarlsberg (my favourite), edam, mascarpone, blue, mozzarella, goats, parmesan. This doesn't include the very processed cheeses such as cream-cheese spreads. The longer a milk product is aged, the lower its carb count, so aged cheeses are great, but not one-month-old milk – that's horrible. Be careful with milk and yoghurt because the high milk sugars in them can still spike your insulin if you are very sensitive to them (see my chapter on plateaus for more about dairy). Also, remember that this is a high-fat, low-carb, *moderate* protein way of eating, so don't go too crazy on cheese. Cottage cheese and ricotta are problematic because they are easy to overeat; for example, a cup of ricotta has 7 grams of carbs, so less is more. You don't have to be wary of butter, though: 10 grams of butter has 8 grams of fat, 0.1 grams of carbs and 0.1 grams of protein. I put it on practically everything. Go for unsalted butter because the salt in salted butter is not sea salt or rock salt. We need salt – we would die without it – but sea salt and rock salt are far better than table salt. Natural salt is 84 per cent sodium chloride, and table salt is 98 per cent. The other 16 per cent in natural salt is chock full of minerals, but the 2 per cent left of table salt is mostly moisture absorbents. To be avoided.

Nuts

Some nuts are better than others. The three best are Brazils, macadamias and pecans. Macadamias are my favourite, with a gorgeous 76 per cent fat content. Hazelnuts, walnuts, pine nuts and almonds are not as good as the top three because their carb count is higher. Run screaming from pistachios (18 grams of carbs per 100 grams) and cashews (27 grams of carbs per 100 grams). A Harvard study into the results from nearly 120,000 participants in the Nurses' Health Study found that daily nut eaters were less likely to die of cancer, heart disease and respiratory disease. The daily nut eaters were overall 20 per cent less likely to have died from anything during the course of the thirty-year study than those who avoided nuts. So, go nuts!

Seeds

Whoa there, Nelly! If most seed oils are bad, why are seeds good? Seeds are a whole unprocessed food that hasn't been subjected to high levels of heating or chemicals to refine it down to an oil. Seeds also contain fibre, minerals and vitamins, plus it is hard to overeat them. The seeds to eat are chia, flax, pumpkin, safflower, sesame and sunflower. Try to buy them raw and whole and not pre-ground because they can go rancid very quickly once they're ground. If you love them ground, use a coffee grinder to grind them at home just before you use them.

The sometimes foods

This is where people trip up on LCHF. I know I did. This is a pretty standard list of the sometimes foods but you will develop your own as you learn which foods trigger cravings for you (for example, I am fine with peanut butter, which is a no-no food, but not fine with too much dairy, as I discovered near the end of my journey). There will also be foods that you will need to put on your own sometimes list if you go to eat a few then find yourself eating fistfuls.

Berries

Okay in moderation, if you are not being very strict or aren't sensitive to their sweetness. Great with Greek yoghurt, whipped cream (not from a can!), mascarpone cheese or a big dollop of double cream. If giving up desserts is your hardest struggle, a handful of berries and some cream after dinner may be your answer. By berries I mean raspberries, strawberries, blackberries, blueberries and cranberries. Of these, choose cranberries and blueberries last. Cranberries have 8 grams of net carbs per 100 grams, and blueberries have a whopping 12, as opposed to the other three, which have 5–6 grams. Always choose fresh, not dried, because the drying process removes the water and concentrates the sugars. And never eat berries canned in sugar syrup.

Vegetables

Watch out for the starchy vegetables such as carrots, parsnips, pumpkin and sweet potato, and only have them sometimes. Also go easy on leeks, tomatoes and onions because they have a slightly higher carb count than most vegies. I find tomatoes very sweet, which can trigger my sweet tooth, so they're something I need to be careful of.

Milk

I know I said full-fat milk was okay but you need to watch the amount you have daily. If you have very milky coffee or tea, this is going to add up over a day and be a problem, not just for carbs but for the milk sugars that can spike your cravings. Try cream in your coffee or cut down on how many cups you have. Anything over 1 cup of milk per day is probably too much and may be the culprit if you are plateauing. I pour my cup of milk out first thing in the morning and fill up my dandelion coffee from that amount and once it's gone for the day it's gone.

Fruit

Why is fruit on the sometimes list when it's natural and unprocessed? Because of fructose. Modern fruit has been developed to be very sweet and is chockful of fructose, which is a sugar. I'm not saying you can't ever eat fruit – fruit *is* a part of this way of eating – just be careful with it. The list below gives you the lowest carbs to the highest, to help you choose the best fruits to eat in moderation. The serving size is a medium piece or a wedge. As you will see, an apricot or a handful of cherries is much better for you than a huge banana.

Fruit	Carbs
Cherry	1
Grape	1
Apricot	3
Lemon	3
Coconut	3
Cantaloupe	5
Plum	7
Peach	8
Pineapple	9
Kiwi	9
Nectarine	12
Orange	12
Honeydew melon	15
Apple	16
Grapefruit	18
Pear	20
Papaya	24
Banana	24
Mango	31

You can see that one pear alone will use up all your carbs for the day if you are on a strict regime.

The never foods

Let's start with the main foods that should never pass your lips. They are: Potatoes, Grains, Sugar, Legumes, Corn, Bad Oils and Processed Foods. That sounds like a lot to remember when looking through a list of ingredients or a restaurant menu, so I've created a little saying to help: Pigs (potatoes) Get (grains) Super (sugar) Levels (legumes) of Control (corn) But Only (bad oils) when Pigs Fly (processed foods).

Okay it's not a brilliant saying, and I'm not suggesting you or anyone else is a pig, but I hope that by the time you remember what each word stands for you will have overlooked the corn fritters on toast and ordered the poached eggs, sautéed mushrooms and avocado without toast and will be flying as free as a bird (pig).

Here is a more detailed list of the foods you will never eat again.

Potatoes

In any way, shape or form. Sebago, dutch creams, kipfler, pontiac, russet and every other type. Why? Because they are high in starch and starch equals sugar. Mashed, baked or cut into chips and wedges, they are a no-no. And don't get me started on potato chips made from a sludge of rice, corn, wheat and potato flakes – all cheap ingredients on the no-no list and, yes, I used the word sludge. Sure, baked potatoes in their skins are better than eating a chocolate bar and their sugar will hit your blood stream slower than the bar will, but they will still spike your insulin, so don't touch them. If potatoes are your absolute favourite food and you can't live without them, don't panic. You can have them occasionally when you lose weight. And by then you might be so in love with fried Brussels sprouts that you might not want potatoes ever

161

again. Trust me on this. As you lose weight you can still occasionally have sweet potato if you are desperate for potato-ness.

Grains

And I mean all grains, even wholegrains. For a start very few foods are actually fully wholegrain. They usually only contain a tiny handful of wholegrains so the manufacturer can put the words 'wholegrain goodness' on the label alongside a picture of a kernel of wheat. Don't be fooled. That wholegrain bread or wholegrain breakfast cereal is full of rice flour, wheat flour, corn and/or sugar. And even if it is fully wholegrain then it will still spike your insulin, and we don't want that. You will get plenty of fibre from eating lots of vegetables and some fruit. You don't need grains of any kind. Speaking of kinds of grains, here is the list to avoid: spelt, quinoa, buckwheat, amaranth, maize, couscous, teff, wheat, rye, millet, barley, sorghum, oats, rice. Don't eat these or their flours or products made from them. So, no rice crackers, porridge, corn thins, spelt bread, etcetera.

Sugar

Avoid all sugar in all its different forms and fancy sciencey names. And sugar is in everything. Did you know that barbecue sauce has more sugar in it than chocolate topping? This is one of the reasons why we only eat real foods. Packaged food is full of sugar. Don't touch fizzy drinks, chocolate bars, cakes, buns, breakfast cereals of any type, ice-cream, frozen yoghurts, flavoured yoghurts, pastries and candy. If in doubt, read the label. Again, not that you are eating anything in a wrapper, but in case you are tempted to, do know that manufacturers have come up with over sixty different names for sugar so they can list them separately on the label and make it look like there is less sugar in it. The main names for sugar are sucrose, fructose, high-fructose corn syrup, barley malt, dextrose, maltose, rice syrup, honey, agave, caramel and molasses. Some Banting/LCHF programs say you can have natural sweeteners such as stevia. I disagree with this for people with a weight problem. You need to lose your sweet tooth, and I don't think using 'better' sweeteners will help that. I now find tomatoes and carrots insanely sweet. The idea of eating a Magnum ice-cream with five teaspoons of sugar in it makes me feel queasy. If you need something sweet have mascarpone cheese or double cream and berries. But not too much and try to wean yourself off this as a regular daily item.

Legumes

But surely legumes are good for you? They are a real food. Hippies eat lentils. Sorry but no, apart from the fact that legumes can be very hard to digest for some people, they are very high in carbs. So, no green peas, chickpeas, lentils, dried beans, peanuts including in the form of peanut butter (the peanut is a starchy legume not a nut) and no soy. What? Soy is healthy, isn't it? Actually, no it isn't. It suppresses thyroid function, which is a good reason not to eat it, but it is also very high in carbs: 100 grams of soybeans contain 30 grams of carbs, which is way too much if you want to be healthy and lose weight.

Corn

Dried corn, or maize, is a grain but I am going to treat it separately because fresh corn is a vegetable and corn is everywhere and you need to watch out for it. A hundred grams of corn has a whopping 74 grams of carbs. And the more you refine corn, such as grind it and make it into a flour, the higher the carb count goes. Maize flour, corn starch and high-fructose corn syrup are very cheap to

produce and can be found in many processed foods. Run screaming to the hills if anyone offers you something with corn in it.

Bad Oils

Back in the seventies, when we were told not to eat fat because
it was supposedly bad for us, we were also told to eat margarine
and seed oils because they were supposedly good. Margarine was
invented in France by Hippolyte Mège-Mouriès in 1869, during the
Franco–Prussian wars, because Napoleon III offered a huge prize
to anyone who could come up with a cheap, stable butter substitute
for French troops to carry as they marched across Europe. So, it's
a cheap version of butter. It is made from seed oils – and that's the
bad part. Most things called vegetable oils are actually seed oils.
These are soybean oil, corn oil, sesame oil, grapeseed oil, peanut oil,
cottonseed oil and sunflower oil. The way these oils are produced
involves a harsh and very modern extraction process that includes
refining, degumming, bleaching and deodorizing, chemicals such
as acid and the highly toxic solvent hexane and heating the oil to
over 250 degrees Celsius. Most oils go rancid after heating to about
50 degrees Celsius. But along with the rancidity and the chemicals
and the bleaching, these oils are also very high in Omega-6 polyun-
saturated fatty acids. Omega-6 isn't toxic so long as it is in balance
with Omega-3s. But eating so much vegetable oil has pushed this
balance out to where some people's diets are as high as 16:1 in favour
of Omega-6. Omega-6 fatty acids build up in our cell membranes
and cause inflammation, which is a factor in diseases such as
cardiovascular disease, cancer, diabetes, arthritis and Alzheimer's.
But wait, there's more! These oils can contain high levels of trans-
fats that are associated with an increased risk of heart attack and
heart disease. Moreover, some of these oils have low smoke points –
the temperature at which an oil starts to smoke and actually breaks

down and releases free radicals – which means they shouldn't be cooked with. The only seed oil to use occasionally for cooking is rice bran oil because it has a very high smoke point, but always buy it in a dark container and not clear plastic because light will make it go rancid. Aprille recommends you vary your cooking oil between butter (270 degrees Celsius smoke point), coconut oil (177), ghee (252) and rice bran oil (254). Extra-virgin olive oil has a smoke point of 160 and is a great oil, she advises, but best added after cooking or on a salad. And you even have to watch out for olive oil because it is often sold as pure but is actually a blend of olive and cheaper seed oils. If it doesn't solidify in the fridge, or isn't from a single farm label or is on special and way too cheap, it is probably an unhealthy blend.

Processed Foods

Do I really need to say anything here? If it's in a box, a carton or a pack you should avoid it. There are some exceptions, such as meat and vegetable stocks. I don't always make my own stock. But this is where you read the packet very carefully. Stocks such as Campbell's chicken stock contain the following: water, chicken, carrot, celery, cabbage, onion, sage extract, parsley, salt, sugar and yeast extract. There are two no-nos on that list: sugar and the yeast extract, which is wheat-based. When I can't be bothered making stock from scratch I buy a very natural range from the health-food section of the supermarket that contains water, meat, salt and pepper and a few vegies such as onions and carrots.

What to drink

Obviously not liquid sugar like Coke, Pepsi, Fanta or sports drinks. Alcohol is a problem too and not just because it relaxes your focus and control. If you need a drink go for a dry white or red wine, dry champagne or the purest of alcohols such as whisky, brandy, gin and vodka. If you are having a cocktail make sure it is made without sugar or fruit juice, and avoid beer. What you can drink is water and lots of it, which is what we should all be having as our main libation anyway. Other things you can drink are tea and coffee (just watch the milk content), herbal teas (make sure they are made without sugar) and coffee substitutes such as dandelion coffee (but watch out for Caro and other coffee substitutes because they often contain barley). Aprille introduced me to soda water and it is my new best friend. It's like having a party in your mouth. We even bought a SodaStream because we all now drink so much of it. She highly recommends a glass of soda water with a dash of apple cider vinegar once a day to help with cravings and to help prevent insulin spiking.

Chapter Sixteen

How many carbs should you eat per day?

Low-carb high-fat is *not* no carb. You eat lots of good carbs, you just get them mostly from leafy greens and other vegetables.

Depending on how much weight you have to lose, how fast you want to lose it and how strict you want to be, here are the guidelines to help you.

Strict: under 20 grams of carbs per day.
Moderate: 20–50 grams of carbs per day.
Go crazy: 50–100 grams of carbs per day.

Some points to remember:

• When you are counting the carbs in a particular food the net carb count is what you are after, not the total carbs. This is because our bodies don't digest the fibre in foods the same way, so it doesn't spike our insulin and therefore doesn't need to be counted. This also means that foods such as high-fibre vegetables have a low carb count and we can eat them happily.

- For the first few weeks or even months use an online food diary to track your net carbs per day to find the level that suits you. If you are plateauing or even putting weight on, go back to the diary to find those sneaky carbs that are tripping you up.
- Going strict low carb will result in faster weight loss but might be harder to sustain. I ate mostly in the upper end of the moderate level and lost weight more slowly than I could have but found this more sustainable and easier to stick to.
- The go-crazy level is more for when you have lost your weight and are in maintenance mode. It's also good for those days when your car won't start or when you get home from work and the kids announce, 'We made a big mess but it's okay, we've cleaned it up!' You know those days. You won't lose weight in this range but some days you just need an extra handful of nuts and an extra serve of konjac carbonara. Don't beat yourself up.
- Everyone is different and everyone's body is different. Experiment with which level works for you.

How many kilojoules (or calories) should you eat?

This way of eating isn't about counting every single kilojoule you put in your mouth. But you can overeat on Banting/LCHF and, if you do, you won't lose weight. If you overeat a lot, you can even put weight on. First of all you need to work out how many kilojoules you should eat per day to maintain your weight. To do this, jump online and search for a free Recommended Daily Intake (RDI) calculator. It will ask your gender, age, weight and height to first work out your Basal Metabolic Rate – the minimal amount of kilojoules your body needs to function if you were at rest all day long.

That's the energy you need to run your organs and breathe and think. Then it will ask for your average level of daily activity (sedentary, slightly active, moderately active, very active). Very active is if you work all day as a dog-walker then run around after quintuplet toddlers all weekend. Few people are very active. The calculator will then tell you how many kilojoules or calories you need each day to function. An average woman is about 8300 kilojoules (2000 calories), and an average man is 10,500 kilojoules (2500 calories). Mine is 8000 kilojoules (1900 calories) because I'm kind of old and you need less as you age.

Don't tape this amount to your fridge or your forehead, just be aware of it and if you have a plateau do an online food diary to measure how many kilojoules you are eating in an average day and make adjustments to be below your RDI. Not 1000 kilojoules below, that's a starvation diet; just a bit below every day so your body can use up your fat stores.

Chapter Seventeen

How to stock your pantry

Aprille says healthy people have a full fridge and an empty pantry, because fresh healthy food goes off.

During our first session she checked my pantry. It was five shelves groaning with packets of food. Then she checked the fridge: a few sad vegetables, some science experiments growing mould and lots of cheese. The only thing she was okay about was the cheese.

Now my pantry is one shelf. Yes, one shelf. The other shelves contain a multitude of containers to carry leftovers to work. The fridge, on the other hand, is a different matter. We play a constant game of Tetris trying to fit food into it.

Here's a list of everyday staples to give you an idea of what to keep on hand. You will develop your own 'must have' list according to the foods you like.

Pantry

Tins of tuna and sardines in olive oil

Konjac noodles – fettucine, rice, lasagne sheets, spaghetti and
angel hair (see page 227)

Jars of passata sauce (tomato pasta sauce without sugar or
anything else in it)

Tins of tomatoes (BPA free)

Rice bran oil (in a tin, not in clear plastic)

Coconut oil

Extra-virgin pressed expensive olive oil (100 per cent pure,
not a cheap brand that is probably a blend of olive oil and
vegetable oil)

Tea

Sesame seeds

Flax seeds

Sunflower seeds

Vinegar

Good quality chicken and beef stock

Almond flour

Coconut flour

Coconut milk

Coconut cream

Apple cider vinegar

Tahini (great on steamed vegetables)

Fridge

Eggs

Butter, unsalted

Full-fat milk

Full-fat Greek yoghurt

Cream (normal cream, sour cream and/or double cream)

Vegetables, so many lovely vegetables

Salad makings

Sweet potato (but only occasionally)

Bacon

Olives

Tamari sauce (fine to keep in the pantry but it retains its flavour for longer if stored in the fridge)

Dijon mustard

Cheeses (notice the plural)

Coffee

Meat, fish and chicken

Occasional punnets of berries

Kitchen bench

Onions

Garlic

Avocadoes

Fresh tomatoes

Nuts

Lemons

A pumpkin occasionally

Himalayan rock salt or sea salt

Herbs and spices

Of course there are things in our cupboard and fridge that I don't eat, such as the sourdough bread that Russell now loves, cacao powder to make hot chocolates for the kids, Vegemite and some flour for making pancakes for the kids and their friends, but I didn't want to clutter the list with those because they might be confusing for you. Pancakes – did she say I could have pancakes?! No, sorry, I didn't. They're for the kids. Have them occasionally when you lose weight and use gluten-free flour and serve them with butter not maple syrup. Yes, I'm a killjoy.

Chapter Eighteen

Aprille's recipes and meal plans

Here are some of my favourite recipes and meal plans that will help you get started. They are just a guide and meals can be swapped around to suit your personal tastes. When I see people in my clinic, I modify these plans depending on what each person's goals are and how rapidly they want to lose weight. This plan is about good health, and when you eat well you naturally lose weight. This isn't about excluding foods that are good for you, some of them just have a time and place. Enjoy, go well and good health!

Aprille McMahon

Aprille's Seed Mix

Serves 8–10

Ingredients

150 grams almond slivers

150 grams chia seeds

150 grams linseeds/flaxseeds

150 grams organic desiccated coconut

150 grams pumpkin seeds

150 grams sesame seeds

150 grams sunflower seeds

100 grams sultanas or raisins or cranberries (this is a very small
amount of fruit for the 1 kilogram of seed mix)

Milk as required

Yoghurt if required

Method

Combine all of the dry ingredients and store in an airtight
container in the cupboard or fridge.

To make one serving soak ½ cup of the seed mix in a cup of
milk overnight. Refrigerate in either a container with a lid or in
a covered bowl. The milk should cover the seed mix by 2cm.

In the morning, the milk will have been absorbed. Add more
milk to taste, or a spoonful of yoghurt.

Note: The seed mix does not have to be soaked overnight, it can
be eaten as is with milk or yoghurt.

Asian Lettuce Cups

Serves 4–6

Ingredients
2 tablespoons olive oil or coconut oil
3 cloves garlic, finely chopped
2-centimetre cube of ginger, finely chopped
2 carrots, thinly sliced
1 tablespoon peanut oil
1 tablespoon sesame oil
salt and pepper, to season
300 grams minced beef
300 grams minced pork
3 tablespoons soy sauce
1 spring onion, chopped
½ cup chopped coriander (more if you like)
cos lettuce
½ cup chopped peanuts, if desired

Method
In a large frying pan, heat the olive oil or coconut oil over a medium heat. Add the garlic, ginger, carrot, peanut oil and sesame oil, season with salt and pepper and mix. Add the mince and combine, cooking until brown. Add the soy sauce and spring onion, and stir.

When serving onto lettuce cups, sprinkle with coriander and peanuts as desired.

Store washed lettuce cups in the fridge until ready to use to ensure crispness.

Beef Burger

Makes 12   Makes 12

Ingredients

Version 1   **Version 2 (fructose friendly)**

butter, for frying   1 kilogram minced beef

½ onion, finely chopped   ½ teaspoon Himalayan salt

3 cloves garlic, finely chopped   ¾ cup grated cheese

2-centimetre cube of ginger,   1 egg
  finely chopped   black pepper, to taste

1 kilogram minced beef

¼ teaspoon black pepper

½ teaspoon Himalayan salt

1 cup grated hard cheese

1 egg

Method

Melt 1 tablespoon of butter in a frying pan over a medium heat
and add the onion, garlic and ginger. Fry until soft and slightly
brown. Remove from heat and set aside until the mixture is cool
enough to handle.

In a large bowl, add all the ingredients, and mix by hand until
well combined.

Use an egg ring to shape the hamburgers (they will not need
to be cooked in the egg rings, this is just to ensure consistency
of size).

In a large frying pan, melt butter and then cook the hamburgers
over a medium heat until golden brown and cooked through –
approximately 5 minutes each side.

Serve with salad or vegetables.

Chicken and Vegetable Fritters

Makes 6

Ingredients

butter, for frying

1 large free-range chicken fillet, finely chopped

2 broccoli heads or the equivalent quantity of mixed vegetables
(to your liking), finely chopped

½ cup pine nuts

5 eggs, beaten

¼ cup parsley, finely chopped

2 cloves garlic, finely chopped

80 grams feta cheese

salt and pepper, to season

100 grams buckwheat flour or coconut flour

Method

In a large frying pan, melt 1–2 tablespoons of butter, then add
the chicken pieces. Cook over a medium heat, turning, for
8 minutes until brown and cooked through. Remove from heat
and set the chicken aside.

Steam the vegetables in a bamboo or metal steamer (with lid)
sitting over a saucepan until soft but not mushy, then shake off
any excess water and set aside in a large, clean bowl.

Place a clean, dry frying pan over medium heat and add the
pine nuts (use a little butter if you like). Fry until the nuts are
brown (watch them carefully as this happens very quickly), then
remove from heat and add to the vegetables.

Add the beaten egg, parsley, garlic and feta to the chicken
and vegetables, combine and season with salt and pepper. Add
the flour gradually, stirring to combine. (You might not need the

whole 100 grams; it is there as a binder. The consistency of the mixture should allow you to make it into a patty without falling apart.) Add the cooked chicken, and combine.

Using your hands, form the batter into palm-size balls then flatten a little; the mixture should make eight. Heat butter over a medium heat in a large frying pan and add the fritters in batches (you might need to add more butter with each batch). Cook the fritters for approximately 5 minutes each side or until cooked through and golden.

Serve with salad or 1½ cups of vegetables.

Chicken on Cauliflower Mash

Serves 4–6

Ingredients

1 tablespoon butter or coconut oil, for frying

1–2 onions, finely chopped (eliminate for a fructose-friendly version)

1 garlic clove, crushed

1 red capsicum, finely chopped

handful green beans, cut in half, ends trimmed

15-centimetre piece sweet potato or 3 carrots, finely chopped

2 tomatoes (optional), finely chopped

1 teaspoon Himalayan salt

1 teaspoon paprika

pepper, to taste

1 kilogram chicken fillets cut into pieces (skin on is fine if you like it)

1 cauliflower, florets finely chopped

butter, for mashing

salt, to season

1 spring onion (green part only for a fructose-friendly version), thinly
  sliced, to serve

Method

Chicken

In a large deep frying pan, melt butter or oil over medium heat.
Add the onion and garlic, and cook until soft.

Add the capsicum, beans and sweet potato or carrot (and
tomatoes), stir to combine, and add the salt and paprika, then
season with pepper and stir-fry for 2 minutes.

Add the chicken and stir-fry, stirring frequently, for
3 minutes.

Cover the chicken with water (don't overdo it, you can add

more if needed). Increase the heat and bring to the boil, then reduce the heat and simmer for 7 minutes until the chicken is cooked through.

Cauliflower mash
While the chicken is simmering, steam the cauliflower in a microwave or on the stove top until soft. Place in a large bowl or food proccessor and mash with butter and some salt to season.

Place the mash on serving plates and cover with a ladle of the chicken pieces and juice. Garnish with the spring onion to serve.

Chicken Schnitzel and Chicken Nuggets

Serves 6

Ingredients

1 egg, beaten

3 free-range chicken breasts, cut in half

½ cup Cornflakes crumbs from the supermarket (it looks like a box of
   breadcrumbs) or crush your own

¼ teaspoon Himalayan salt

pepper, to taste

½ teaspoon oregano

Plus any other spices you might like to add to the crumb mix

olive oil or butter, for frying

Method

For schnitzel

Place the beaten egg in a shallow bowl, then add the chicken and
coat the chicken with egg.

Put ½ cup of the Cornflakes crumbs (more or less depending
on how much chicken you are using) in a shallow bowl, then
add the salt, pepper, oregano and any other spices.

Add one piece of chicken at a time and coat with the crumbs,
then transfer to a plate. Repeat until all the chicken is coated. (If
you are not cooking the chicken straightaway, store in the fridge.)

Melt oil or butter in a large frying pan over medium heat.
Add the schnitzel and fry, checking regularly, until just cooked.
(The more it is cooked the less tender it will be.)

For nuggets
Cut the chicken into smaller pieces, follow the crumbing and cooking process for schnitzel, then serve both with 1½ cups of salad or vegetables.

Note: If you like to eat schnitzel, Cornflakes, while high GI, processed and containing sugar, are still a better option than breadcrumbs because they are wheat-free. It's not ideal, I know, but it's okay once in a while – and it's better than traditional schnitzel. You can also experiment with almond meal instead.

Egg Salad

Serves 1

Ingredients

Salad

2 eggs, hard-boiled and cooled, then peeled and chopped

½ carrot, grated

¼ Lebanese cucumber, chopped

¼ red capsicum, finely chopped

2 mushrooms, sliced

5 baby tomatoes, halved

½ avocado, finely chopped

handful baby spinach leaves

Dressing

2 tablespoons extra-virgin olive oil

pinch of Himalayan salt

pinch of pepper

¼ teaspoon turmeric

1 tablespoon lemon juice

¼ teaspoon oregano (dried or fresh is fine)

Method

Combine all the salad ingredients in a large bowl. Combine all the dressing ingredients in a jug, and drizzle the dressing over the salad to serve.

Frittata

Serves 4–6

Ingredients

coconut oil, ghee or butter, to stir-fry the vegetables

2–3 cups vegetables of your choice, to stir-fry

3 rashers bacon, finely chopped

1 onion, finely chopped (remove for a fructose-friendly version)

10 eggs

½ teaspoon Himalayan salt

pepper, to season

1 cup grated cheese, plus extra cheese for the top of the frittata

½–1 cup chopped parsley (optional)

2 cups baby spinach leaves

Method

Preheat oven to 180 degrees (160 degrees fan-forced).

In a large frying pan, melt the oil, ghee or butter over medium heat. Add the vegetables and cook, stirring, until cooked but still crunchy. Remove the vegetables from the pan and set aside to cool.

Add the bacon and onion to the frying pan and cook, stirring, until golden. Return the cooked vegetables to the pan and stir to combine. Remove from the heat and set aside.

In a large bowl, beat the eggs. Season with the salt and pepper, and add any other spices you like to the egg mix. Add the vegetables and bacon from the frying pan and stir to combine, then add the grated cheese and parsley, and again stir to combine.

In a round silicon oven-proof flan dish (approximately 26 centimetres in diameter), place the baby spinach leaves at the bottom. Pour the egg and vegetable mix over the spinach, then sprinkle extra cheese over the top so that the mix is covered.

Cook for 30 minutes or until the top is golden brown.

Serve with a salad or vegetables.

Lamb Burgers

Makes 9

Ingredients

1 medium-sized sweet potato, approximately 250 grams, peeled and
 chopped

butter, for mashing

1 onion, finely chopped (optional – remove for a fructose-friendly
 version)

500 grams lamb mince

1 egg, beaten

1 carrot, grated (optional)

1 zucchini, grated (optional)

garlic, crushed (optional, to taste)

ginger, finely chopped or grated (optional, to taste)

½ teaspoon Himalayan salt

pepper, to season

butter, for frying

Greek yoghurt (optional)

Method

Bring a saucepan of water to the boil and add the sweet potato.
Allow to boil for 15 minutes or until soft, then remove from
the heat and drain. Add butter and mash the sweet potato until
smooth, then set aside and allow to cool.

 While the sweet potato is cooling, add a little butter to a small
sauté pan and melt over medium heat. Add the onion and cook,
stirring, until the onion is soft. Remove from the heat and set
aside.

 In a bowl, add the mince, egg, carrot, zucchini, garlic and
ginger, then season with the salt and pepper and stir to combine

well. (If time permits, put the mixture in the fridge or freezer for 30 minutes to bind it well.)

Use an egg ring to shape the burgers (they will not need to be cooked in the egg rings, this is just to ensure consistency of size).

In a large pan, melt the butter and then cook the burgers over a medium heat until golden brown and cooked through – approximately 5 minutes each side.

Put a dollop of Greek yoghurt on each burger when serving (optional) with salad or vegetables.

Lamb Shoulder with Gravy and Vegetables

Serves 6–8

Ingredients

1.5–2-kilogram lamb shoulder (boneless)

olive oil

salt and pepper, to season

fresh rosemary

vegetables for roasting, chopped (choose vegetables you like but try to avoid potato and corn because these are high GI)

1–1½ cups chicken stock (use homemade or a Banting-friendly option – see page 165. You can also use a preservative-free stock powder such as Massel)

2–3 tablespoons gluten-free plain flour

Method

Preheat oven to 150 degrees (130 degrees fan-forced).

Place the lamb shoulder on a baking tray and baste with the olive oil, and season with salt and pepper. Poke some rosemary sprigs into the shoulder, evenly spaced.

Cook at 130 degrees Celsius for 4 hours. When ready, the lamb should fall apart and be so soft that it is difficult to cut. Season with salt and pepper to taste before serving with the vegetables and gravy.

About an hour before the lamb is ready start doing the vegetables. Place the roast on the bottom of the oven and use a different tray to roast the vegetables in the middle of the oven.

Place vegetables in the roasting tray, drizzle with olive oil and toss to ensure they are evenly coated. Cook them in stages depending on what type of vegetable they are. Firmer, thicker vegetables will need to be cooked for longer – around an hour for potato and pumpkin. Sweet potato, carrot, pumpkin, beans, onion and mushrooms work well with a roast.

When the lamb is cooked, remove it from the oven and wrap it in foil and two tea towels and allow to rest for 30 minutes.

Keep the juices in the pan ready to make the gravy.

Gravy

When you are ready to make the gravy, place the oven tray with pan juices on the stove over a medium heat and begin to warm it. Add the stock and stir well with a wooden spoon as it heats. Gradually add the flour and mix well. (Add more or less flour depending on how thick you would like it to be.)

When you transfer the gravy into a gravy boat, skim any fat from the top and keep it in a container to use to fry other things later in the week.

Lamb with Coconut Cream

Serves 4–6

Ingredients

coconut oil, butter or ghee, for frying

1 kilogram diced lamb

800 grams tinned diced tomatoes

water as required

1 onion (remove for a fructose-friendly version)

2 cloves garlic, crushed (remove for a fructose-friendly version)

ginger, finely chopped or grated

salt and pepper, to season

140 millilitres coconut cream (full fat)

3 cups of vegetables of your choice, chopped into small pieces (green
   beans, capsicum, broccoli, cauliflower, zucchini or carrot are all good)

Method

This recipe will take up to 1½ hours to cook. This will ensure
that the meat becomes nice and tender. Test it as you go.

In a large frying pan, melt the oil, lard or ghee over a medium
heat. Add the lamb and cook over a medium heat, turning, until
brown.

Add the tomatoes and allow to simmer. When the liquid
begins to reduce, add water periodically so the liquid can reduce
but not dry out.

Add the garlic and ginger, and season with salt and pepper.
Stir, and continue to allow the mixture to simmer and reduce,
adding water when required.

Add the coconut cream in the last 20 minutes of cooking.

You can add the vegetables to the pan or stir-fry them as a side
dish. If you add the vegetables to the pan, time it so that they are
as soft or as crunchy as your family likes them.

Oven-roasted Chicken Drumettes

Serves 6

Ingredients
25 chicken drumettes

Marinade
2 tablespoons lemon juice
½ teaspoon turmeric
1 teaspoon cumin
1 teaspoon Himalayan salt
1 large garlic clove
1-centimetre thick piece of ginger, chopped
olive oil, butter, ghee or coconut oil
pepper, to taste (if desired)

Method
Place the chicken drumettes in a container and set aside.

In a bowl, combine all marinade ingredients and whiz with a handheld blender or in a food processor.

Pour the marinade over the chicken and mix until all the chicken is coated. Place a lid on the container and refrigerate for a minimum of 2 hours, and up to 12 hours.

Preheat oven to 210 degrees (200 degrees fan-forced). Line a baking tray with foil.

Place the chicken in a single layer on the oven tray and then place on a wire rack in the oven. Bake for 25–35 minutes or until well browned and cooked through.

Poached Chicken Breast

Serves 2

Ingredients

2 free-range chicken breasts (alter the amount depending on how many you need to feed), cut into evenly sized pieces

Method

Bring a saucepan of water to the boil, then reduce the heat to low and place the chicken pieces into the water. Poach the chicken until it is just cooked (around 13–15 minutes). Remove from the water and serve with salad or vegetables.

Pulled Pork with Gravy and Vegetables

Serves 6

Ingredients

1½ kilogram pork shoulder/neck (boneless)

olive oil, plus extra to coat the vegetables

salt and pepper, to season

vegetables for roasting (avoid potato and corn because these are high GI)

1–1½ cups chicken stock (use a homemade or a Banting-friendly option – see page 165. You can also use preservative-free stock powder such as Massel)

2–3 tablespoons gluten-free plain flour

Method

Preheat oven to 130 degrees (110 degrees fan-forced).

Pork

Place the pork shoulder on a baking tray and baste with olive oil, salt and pepper. Bake for 5 hours. When ready, the pork should fall apart and be so soft that it is difficult to cut. Season with salt and pepper to taste before serving with the vegetables and gravy.

Vegetables

After the pork has been in the oven for 4 hours you can start doing the vegetables. Place the roast on the bottom of the oven and use a different tray to roast the vegetables in the middle of the oven.

Place vegetables in the roasting tray, drizzle with olive oil and toss to ensure they are evenly coated. Cook them in stages depending on what type of vegetable they are. Sweet potato, carrot, zucchini, broccoli, cauliflower, onion and mushroom are suitable.

When they are cooked, remove them from the oven and wrap them in foil and two tea towels and allow to rest for 30 minutes.

Keep the juices in the pan ready to make the gravy.

Gravy
When you are ready to make the gravy, place the oven tray with pan juices on the stove over a medium heat and begin to warm it. Add the stock and stir well with a wooden spoon as it heats. Gradually add the flour and mix well. (Add more or less flour depending on how thick you would like it to be.)

When you transfer the gravy into a gravy boat, skim any fat from the top and keep it in a container to use to fry other things later in the week.

Pumpkin Soup with Ginger, Coconut and Cashews

Serves 4

Ingredients

½ Jap pumpkin, peeled and chopped into 2-centimetre thick slices

2 tablespoons olive oil

¾ cup cashews (optional)

2-centimetre cube fresh ginger

1 tablespoon coconut oil

½–¾ teaspoon Himalayan salt

¾ teaspoon cumin

¾ teaspoon paprika

20 grams butter

Method

Preheat oven to 220 degrees (210 degrees for fan-forced) and line a baking tray with baking paper.

Place the chopped pumpkin and olive oil in a bowl and toss to combine.

Place the oiled pumpkin onto the tray lined with baking paper and bake for 15–20 minutes or until soft when tested with a fork.

Meanwhile, in a food processor, combine the cashews, ginger and coconut oil until they form a smooth paste.

When the pumpkin is cooked, transfer it to a saucepan over a medium heat with ½ cup of water, then add the cashew and ginger paste as well as the salt, cumin, paprika and butter. Mash the pumpkin and paste until it combines well into a soup consistency. (Add extra water if necessary until you get your preferred consistency.)

Refried Lamb Shoulder with Vegetables and Yoghurt

Serves 4

Ingredients

leftover roast lamb shoulder from previous day, sliced

3 tablespoons coconut oil

3 tablespoons butter or lard for cooking the vegetables

1 eggplant, chopped

1 medium sweet potato, peeled and chopped

100 grams beans, washed and trimmed

1 carrot, peeled and chopped

¼ cauliflower, chopped (stalks removed)

1 medium floret broccoli, chopped (stalks removed)

1 zucchini, chopped

100 grams mushrooms, sliced

1 capsicum, chopped

2 tablespoons Greek yoghurt

Method

Heat the coconut oil in a frying pan over a medium heat, then add the lamb. Once warm, the lamb should break up into small pieces.

While the lamb cooks, heat the butter in a large frying pan over a medium heat. Add the eggplant and sweet potato and stir-fry until they soften, then remove them from the pan and set them aside. If necessary add more butter to the pan and then add the remaining vegetables and stir-fry until they are soft, then remove them from the heat and add to the eggplant and sweet potato.

Serve lamb with 1½ cups of the vegetables and Greek yoghurt.

Salmon Salad

Serves 2

Ingredients

100 grams cooked salmon, flaked

1 large handful rocket leaves (or other leaf if you prefer)

2 tablespoons sunflower seeds

2 tablespoons pumpkin seeds

½ avocado, chopped

2 tablespoons olive oil or avocado oil

salt and pepper, to season

Method

In a large bowl, combine all the ingredients, then season with salt to serve.

Shepherd's Pie with Cauliflower Mash

Serves 4–6

This recipe uses a 32-centimetre rectangular casserole dish

Ingredients

olive oil, coconut oil or butter, for frying

1 brown onion, peeled and finely chopped (remove to make a fructose-friendly version)

Meat and vegetable base

500 grams minced beef

500 grams minced lamb

140 grams (1½ cups) tomato paste

1 teaspoon cumin

2 teaspoons curry powder

1 teaspoon Himalayan salt

½ capsicum, finely chopped

1 stick celery, finely chopped

10 green beans, trimmed and chopped

2 carrots, peeled and finely chopped

And any other vegetables you like

Cauliflower mash topping

1½–2 cauliflowers, chopped (stalks removed)

1–2 tablespoons butter

1 cup grated cheese

1 teaspoon salt

Method

Preheat oven to 180 degrees (160 degrees fan-forced).

In a large frying pan, heat the oil or butter over a medium heat, then add the onion and cook until soft. Add the mince and cook, stirring to mix with the onion until brown. Add the tomato paste, cumin and curry powder and stir to combine. Season with salt.

Meanwhile, in another frying pan, heat the oil or butter over a medium heat, then add the vegetables and stir until cooked through. Combine the vegetables with the meat, and stir to combine. Set aside while you prepare the cauliflower.

Steam the cauliflower until very soft. Place in a large bowl or food processor and mash with the butter and salt. Mix until you achieve your preferred mash consistency.

In a large casserole dish, place the meat/vegetable mix on the bottom, then carefully spoon the cauliflower mash over the top. Finally, sprinkle the grated cheese over the top.

Bake for 30 minutes or until the cheese is melted and as brown as you like it.

Smoothie

Serves 1

Ingredients
2 tablespoons almonds
1 teaspoon cinnamon
1 tablespoon chia seeds
1 teaspoon coconut oil
1 tablespoon oats (this is on the never list but we are using a small
    amount here to give the drink a thick, creamy texture. By all means
    leave out if you're being strict)
½ cup cream
1 raw egg
½ cup milk (full cream)

Combine all the ingredients in a blender and mix until you
achieve a smoothie consistency.

Stir-fried Vegetables

Serves 4

Ingredients
coconut oil or butter, for frying (plus extra)
1 eggplant, chopped
½ medium sweet potato, peeled and chopped
1 carrot, peeled and chopped
¼ cauliflower, chopped (stalk removed)
1 medium floret broccoli, chopped (stalk removed)
1 zucchini, chopped
1 red capsicum, chopped
100 grams green beans, trimmed and chopped
100 grams mushrooms, sliced
salt and pepper, to season
oregano, to taste
turmeric, to taste
garlic, crushed, to taste (eliminate for a fructose-friendly version)
ginger, finely chopped, to taste

Method
Heat the oil or butter in a large frying pan over medium heat. Add the eggplant and sweet potato and stir-fry until they soften, then remove them from the pan and set them aside. If necessary add more oil or butter to the pan and then add the carrot, cauliflower, broccoli and zucchini and stir-fry until they are soft. Add the capsicum, beans and mushrooms and stir-fry, taking care not to overcook these last vegetables. When they are almost cooked, add 1 tablespoon of coconut oil to the vegetables and mix well. Season with salt and pepper and add your preferred quantities of oregano, turmeric, garlic and ginger. Remove from heat and serve.

Stuffed Capsicums

Serves 4–5

Ingredients
butter, for frying
1 brown onion, peeled and finely chopped (remove for a
   fructose-friendly version)
500 grams minced beef
1 zucchini, finely chopped
2 carrots, peeled and finely chopped
1 handful green beans, trimmed and finely chopped
1 teaspoon chicken stock powder (use a preservative-free stock
   powder such as Massel)
1 tablespoon Middle Eastern spice mix
2 cloves garlic, crushed
1 teaspoon Himalayan salt
pepper, to season
4–5 large capsicums halved and seeded
Greek yoghurt, to serve
coriander, chopped, to serve
finely grated zest of 1 lemon, to serve

Method
Preheat oven to 180 degrees (160 degrees fan-forced).

In a large frying pan, heat 1 tablespoon butter, and add the
onion. Cook until soft, then add the mince. Cook, stirring,
until brown.

Add another tablespoon of butter and then add the zucchini,
carrot and beans, and stir to combine. Add the stock powder,
spice mix, garlic and salt, and season with pepper. Stir-fry until
the vegetables are cooked.

Place the capsicum halves on a lined baking tray. Using a spoon, fill each capsicum with the mince mixture. Bake for 20 minutes or until the capsicum has softened. (You may need to cover them with foil after 10 minutes so they don't burn.)

To serve, add a spoonful of yoghurt, chopped coriander and a sprinkle of lemon zest.

Zucchini Pasta with Creamy Prawn Sauce

Serves 3–4

Ingredients

butter, for frying, plus extra for the cream sauce
500–750 grams prawns (raw), shelled and patted dry
¾ cup cream
1 tablespoon basil pesto
salt and pepper, to taste
3 zucchinis

Method

In a large frying pan, heat 2 tablespoons butter over a medium heat and add the prawns (use Australian prawns, as they are healthier and a more sustainable option). Stir until prawns are cooked through, then remove from heat.

In a small frying pan, heat another 2 tablespoons butter until melted, then add the cream and stir for 2 minutes until well combined and beginning to thicken. Add 2 tablespoons of the pesto and stir to combine. Season with salt and pepper to taste, and set aside to serve with the zucchini pasta.

Use a spiraliser or julienne peeler to form the zucchini into spirals.

In a large frying pan, heat 2 tablespoons butter, then add the zucchini. Stir to coat the zucchini with butter, then season with salt and pepper. Cook until slightly tender.

Serve the zucchini pasta topped with the creamy prawn sauce.

Zucchini Pie

Serves 5

Ingredients
10 eggs
1 teaspoon Himalayan salt
pepper, to season
butter, for frying
1 onion, sliced (remove for a fructose-friendly version)
4 zucchinis, sliced
½ cauliflower, finely chopped, stalk removed
1 cup grated tasty cheese
2 handfuls spinach or other green leafy vegetable
1 tomato, sliced (optional)

Method
Preheat oven to 180 degrees (160 degrees fan-forced).
In a large bowl, beat the eggs. Add the salt and season with pepper then set aside.

In a frying pan, heat 1 tablespoon butter over medium heat, and add the onion. Saute until the onion is soft, then add the zucchini and cauliflower. Stir-fry until the vegetables have softened but are not too soft, then remove from heat and transfer to a bowl. Stir in the grated cheese, and add the egg and mix well.

Line a baking dish with the spinach (or other green leafy vegetable). Pour over the egg and vegetables, then top with the tomato slices. Bake for 30 minutes.

Serve with salad.

Week 1 Meal Plan

Monday

Breakfast

½ cup Aprille's Seed Mix (page 175) covered with full-cream milk and soaked overnight in the fridge

Snack

1 serve of fruit (see list)**

Lunch

Egg Salad (page 184)

Snack

1 serve from the alternative snack options (see list)*

Dinner

1 fist-sized portion of white fish (fried or baked) with
1½ cups vegetables or salad

(Fish should be wild-caught, not farmed)

Tuesday

Breakfast

200 grams Greek or plain yoghurt with 2 tablespoons mixed chopped nuts (choose from: almonds, macadamia, pecans, hazelnuts, walnuts)

Snack

1 serve from the alternative snack options (see list)*

Lunch

1 fist-sized portion of white fish (leftovers) with 1 cup of vegetables or salad

Snack

1 serve of fruit (see list)**

Dinner

1 fist-sized portion of Shepherd's Pie with Cauliflower Mash (page 199) with 1½ cups vegetables

Wednesday

Breakfast

Smoothie (page 201), 1 cup

Snack

1 serve of fruit (see list)**

Lunch

1 fist-sized portion of Shepherd's Pie (leftovers) with 1 cup of vegetables or salad

Snack

1 serve from the alternative snack options (see list)*

Dinner

1 fist-sized triangle portion of Frittata (page 185) with 1½ cups vegetables or salad

Thursday

Breakfast

½ cup Aprille's Seed Mix (page 175) covered with full-cream milk and soaked overnight in the fridge

Snack

1 serve from the alternative snack options (see list)*

Lunch

1 fist-sized triangle portion of Frittata (leftovers) with 1 cup vegetables or salad

Snack

1 serve of fruit (see list)**

Dinner

100 grams chicken or Chicken Schnitzel (page 182)
with 1½ cups vegetables or salad

Friday

Breakfast

200 grams Greek or plain yoghurt with 2 tablespoons mixed chopped
nuts (choose from: almonds, macadamia, pecans, hazelnuts, walnuts)

Snack

1 serve of fruit (see list)**

Lunch

1 fist-sized portion of Chicken Schnitzel (leftovers) with
1 cup vegetables or salad

Snack

1 serve from the alternative snack options (see list)*

Dinner

1 fist-sized portion pork steak with 1½ cups vegetables or salad

Saturday

Breakfast

2 eggs with 1½ cups stir-fried vegetables (no bread)

Snack

1 serve from the alternative snack options (see list)*

Lunch

1 fist-sized portion of pork steak (leftovers) with
1 cup vegetables or salad

Snack

1 serve of fruit (see list)**

Dinner

1 fist-sized portion of salmon (fried or baked) with
1½ cups vegetables or salad

Sunday

Breakfast

½ cup Aprille's Seed Mix (page 175) covered with full-cream milk and
soaked overnight in the fridge

Snack

1 serve of fruit (see list)**

Lunch

1 large fist-sized portion or two small Beef Burgers (page 177) with salad

Snack

1 serve from the alternative snack options (see list)*

Dinner

1 fist-sized portion of roast Lamb Shoulder (page 189) with 1½ cup roast
vegetables with homemade gravy

NOTES

<u>Snacks</u>

- Up to 2 snacks per day only
- If you want an after-dinner snack, eat breakfast later in the morning
e.g. 10am, and don't have a morning snack

<u>Oils for salads:</u>

- Olive or avocado

<u>Oils for frying:</u>

- Butter
- Coconut
- Olive

- Ghee
- Rice Bran

<u>Vegetables</u>

- At least 5–6 types at a time
- Examples: zucchini, cauliflower, beans, carrot, mushroom, sweet potato, beetroot, eggplant, Brussels sprouts, spinach, capsicum

---

**1 fruit serving: 4 small apricots, 1 small apple, 1 cup berries, ½ banana, 1 cup fruit salad, 1 cup grapes, 2 kiwifruit, 2 cups diced honeydew melon, 1 small orange, 1 large nectarine, ½ mango, 2 small mandarins, 1 small pear, 1 large peach, 2 rings fresh pineapple (1cm thick), 3 small plums, ½ cup diced rockmelon, 3 watermelon wedges (1cm thick) or 2 cups diced

*Alternative snack options: ¼ cup mixed nuts, 150 grams yoghurt, carrot sticks or other chopped vegetables, 40 grams (2 slices) cheese, 1 boiled egg, 1 x 210ml glass wine (less than a standard cup)

Week 2 Meal Plan

Monday

Breakfast

½ cup Aprille's Seed Mix (page 175) covered with full-cream milk soaked overnight in the fridge

Snack

1 serve of fruit (see list)**

Lunch

1 fist-sized quantity of Lamb Shoulder (leftovers) with 1 cup vegetables or salad

Snack

1 serve from the alternative snack options (see list)*

Snack

Poached Chicken Breast (page 193) with 1½ cups vegetables or salad

Tuesday

Breakfast

200 grams Greek or plain yoghurt with 2 tablespoons mixed chopped nuts (choose from: almonds, macadamia, pecans, hazelnuts, walnuts)

Snack

1 serve from the alternative snack options (see list)*

Lunch

1 fist-sized portion of chicken (leftovers) with 1 cup vegetables or salad

Snack

1 serve of fruit (see list)**

Dinner

1 fist-sized portion of white fish (fried or baked) with
1½ cups vegetables or salad
(Fish should be wild-caught, not farmed)

Wednesday

Breakfast

Smoothie (page 201), 1 cup

Snack

1 serve of fruit (see list)**

Lunch

1 fist-sized portion of fish (leftovers) with 1 cup vegetables or salad

Snack

1 serve from the alternative snack options (see list)*

Dinner

1 fist-sized portion of Shepherd's Pie with Cauliflower Mash (page 199)
and vegetables

Thursday

Breakfast

½ cup Aprille's Seed Mix (page 175) covered with full-cream milk or
cream and soaked overnight in the fridge

Snack

1 serve from the alternative snack options (see list)*

Lunch

1 fist-sized portion of Shepherd's Pie (leftovers) with
1 cup vegetables or salad

Snack

1 serve of fruit (see list)**

Dinner

1 fist-sized portion of Lamb with Coconut Cream (page 191) and
1½ cups vegetables

Saturday

Breakfast

2 eggs with 1½ cups stir-fried vegetables (no bread)

Snack

1 serve from the alternative snack options (see list)*

Lunch

1 fist-sized portion of Chicken Drumettes (page 192) with
1 cup vegetables or salad

Snack

1 serve of fruit (see list)**

Dinner

2 Stuffed Capsicums (page 203) with vegetables

Sunday

Breakfast

½ cup Aprille's Seed Mix (page 175) covered with full-cream milk and
soaked overnight in the fridge

Snack

1 serve of fruit (see list)**

Lunch

1 fist-sized portion of Stuffed Capsicums (leftovers) with 1 cup
vegetables or salad

Snack

1 serve from the alternative snack options (see list)*

Dinner

Fist-sized Pulled Pork with Gravy and Vegetables (page 194)

NOTES

Snacks

- 0–2 snacks per day only
- If you want an after-dinner snack then eat breakfast later in the morning e.g. 10am, and don't have a morning snack

Oils for salads:

- Olive or avocado

Oils for frying:

- Butter
- Coconut
- Olive
- Ghee
- Rice Bran

Vegetables

- At least 5–6 types at a time
- Examples: zucchini, cauliflower, beans, carrot, mushroom, sweet potato, beetroot, eggplant, Brussels sprouts, spinach, capsicum

---

**1 Fruit serving: 4 small apricots, 1 small apple, 1 cup berries, ½ banana, 1 cup fruit salad, 1 cup grapes, 2 kiwifruit, 2 cups diced honeydew melon, 1 small orange, 1 large nectarine, ½ mango, 2 small mandarins, 1 small pear, 1 large peach, 2 rings fresh pineapple (1cm thick), 3 small plums, ½ cup diced rockmelon, 3 watermelon wedges (1cm thick) or 2 cups diced

*Alternative snack options: ¼ cup mixed nuts, 150 grams yoghurt, carrot sticks or other chopped vegetables, 40 grams (2 slices) cheese, 1 boiled egg, 1 x 210ml glass wine (less than a standard cup)

Week 3 Meal Plan

Monday

Breakfast
½ cup Aprille's Seed Mix (page 175) covered with full-cream milk soaked overnight in the fridge

Snack
1 serve of fruit (see list)**

Lunch
1 fist-sized portion of Pulled Pork (leftovers) with
1 cup vegetables or salad

Snack
1 serve from the alternative snack options (see list)*

Dinner
1 fist-sized portion of Chicken Schnitzel (page 182)
with 1½ cups vegetables

Tuesday

Breakfast
200 grams Greek or plain yoghurt with 2 tablespoons mixed chopped nuts (choose from: almonds, macadamia, pecans, hazelnuts, walnuts)

Snack
1 serve from the alternative snack options (see list)*

Lunch
1 fist-sized portion of Chicken Schnitzel (leftovers) with
1 cup vegetables or salad

Snack

1 serve of fruit (see list)**

Dinner

1 fist-sized portion of white fish (fried or baked) with
1½ cups vegetables or salad

(Fish should be wild-caught, not farmed)

Wednesday

Breakfast

Smoothie (page 201), 1 cup

Snack

1 serve of fruit (see list)**

Lunch

1 fist-sized portion of white fish (leftovers) with 1 cup vegetables or salad

Snack

1 serve from the alternative snack options (see list)*

Dinner

1 fist-sized portion of Zucchini Pasta with Creamy Prawn Sauce
(page 205) with 1 cup vegetables or salad

Thursday

Breakfast

½ cup Aprille's Seed Mix (page 175) covered with full-cream milk or
cream and soaked overnight in the fridge

Snack

1 serve from the alternative snack options (see list)*

Lunch

1 fist-sized portion of Zucchini Pasta with Creamy Prawn Sauce
(leftovers) with 1 cup vegetables or salad

Snack

1 serve of fruit (see list)**

Dinner

1 hand-sized triangle portion of Frittata (page 185) with 1½ cups
vegetables or salad

Friday

Breakfast

200 grams Greek or plain yoghurt with 2 tablespoons mixed chopped
nuts (choose from: almonds, macadamia, pecans, hazelnuts, walnuts)

Snack

1 serve of fruit (see list)**

Lunch

1 fist-sized triangle portion of Frittata (leftovers) with 1 cup vegetables
or salad

Snack

1 serve from the alternative snack options (see list)*

Dinner

Asian Lettuce Cups (page 176) – enough lettuce cups to hold 1 cup of
the meat mixture – with 1½ cups vegetables or salad

Saturday

Breakfast

2 eggs with 1½ cups stir-fried vegetables (no bread)

Snack

1 serve from the alternative snack options (see list)*

Lunch

Asian Lettuce Cups (leftovers) with 1 cup vegetables or salad

Snack

1 serve of fruit (see list)**

Dinner

1 palm-sized or 2 small Beef Burgers (page 177) with 1½ cups
vegetables or salad

Sunday

Breakfast

½ cup Aprille's Seed Mix (page 175) covered with full-cream milk
and soaked overnight in the fridge

Snack

1 serve of fruit (see list)**

Lunch

1 fist-sized or 2 small Beef Burgers (leftovers) with
1 cup vegetables or salad

Snack

1 serve from the alternative snack options (see list)*

Dinner

Palm-sized portion of Chicken on Cauliflower Mash (page 180) with
1½ cups vegetables or salad

NOTES

Snacks

- Up to 2 snacks per day only
- If you want an after-dinner snack, eat breakfast later in the morning
e.g. 10am, and don't have a morning snack

Oils for salads:

- Olive or avocado

Oils for frying:

- Butter
- Coconut
- Olive
- Ghee
- Rice Bran

<u>Vegetables</u>

- At least 5–6 types at a time
- Examples: zucchini, cauliflower, beans, carrot, mushroom, sweet potato, beetroot, eggplant, Brussels sprouts, spinach, capsicum

---

**1 Fruit serving: 4 small apricots, 1 small apple, 1 cup berries, ½ banana, 1 cup fruit salad, 1 cup grapes, 2 kiwifruit, 2 cups diced honeydew melon, 1 small orange, 1 large nectarine, ½ mango, 2 small mandarins, 1 small pear, 1 large peach, 2 rings fresh pineapple (1cm thick), 3 small plums, ½ cup diced rockmelon, 3 watermelon wedges (1cm thick) or 2 cups diced

*Alternative snack options: ¼ cup mixed nuts, 150 grams yoghurt, carrot sticks or other chopped vegetables, 40 grams (2 slices) cheese, 1 boiled egg, 1 x 210ml glass wine (less than a standard cup)

Week 4 Meal Plan

Monday

Breakfast

½ cup Aprille's Seed Mix (page 175) covered with full-cream milk soaked overnight in the fridge

Snack

1 serve of fruit (see list)**

Lunch

1 fist-sized portion of chicken on 1 fist-sized portion of cauliflower mash (leftovers) with 1 cup vegetables or salad

Snack

1 serve from the alternative snack options (see list)*

Dinner

1 fist-sized portion of Zucchini Pie (page 206) with 1½ cups vegetables or salad

Tuesday

Breakfast

200 grams Greek or plain yoghurt with 2 tablespoons mixed chopped nuts (choose from: almonds, macadamia, pecans, hazelnuts, walnuts)

Snack

1 serve from the alternative snack options (see list)*

Lunch

1 fist-sized portion of Zucchini Pie (leftovers) with 1 cup vegetables or salad

Snack

1 serve of fruit (see list)**

Dinner

1 fist-sized portion of white fish (fried or baked) with 1½ cups
vegetables or salad
(Fish should be wild-caught, not farmed)

Wednesday

Breakfast

Smoothie (page 201), 1 cup

Snack

1 serve of fruit (see list)**

Lunch

1 fist-sized portion of white fish (leftovers) with
1 cup vegetables or salad

Snack

1 serve from the alternative snack options (see list)*

Dinner

1 fist-sized portion of Lamb Shoulder (page 189) with 1½ cups
vegetables or salad

Thursday

Breakfast

½ cup Aprille's Seed Mix (page 175) covered with full-cream milk or
cream and soaked overnight in the fridge

Snack

1 serve from the alternative snack options (see list)*

Lunch

1 fist-sized portion of Lamb Shoulder (leftovers) with
1 cup vegetables or salad

Snack

1 serve of fruit (see list)**

Dinner
1 palm-sized Beef Burger (page 177) with 1½ cups vegetables or salad

Friday

Breakfast
200 grams Greek or plain yoghurt with 2 tablespoons mixed chopped nuts (choose from: almonds, macadamia, pecans, hazelnuts, walnuts)

Snack
1 serve of fruit (see list)**

Lunch
1 palm-sized Beef Burger (leftovers) with
1 cup vegetables or salad

Snack
1 serve from the alternative snack options (see list)*

Dinner
1 fist-sized portion pork steak with 1½ cups vegetables or salad

Saturday

Breakfast
2 eggs with 1½ cups stir-fried vegetables (no bread)

Snack
1 serve from the alternative snack options (see list)*

Lunch
1 fist-sized portion of pork steak (leftovers) with
1 cup vegetables or salad

Snack
1 serve of fruit (see list)**

Dinner

1 fist-sized portion of white fish (fried or baked) with
1½ cups vegetables or salad
(Fish should be wild-caught, not farmed)

Sunday

Breakfast

½ cup Aprille's Seed Mix (page 175) covered with full-cream milk soaked
overnight in the fridge

Snack

1 serve of fruit (see list)**

Lunch

One large fist-sized portion of white fish (leftovers) with 1 cup vegetables
or salad

Snack

1 serve from the alternative snack options (see list)*

Dinner

1 fist-sized portion of Poached Chicken Breast (page 193) with
1½ cups of vegetables or salad

NOTES

Snacks

- Up to 2 snacks per day only
- If you want an after-dinner snack, eat breakfast later in the morning
e.g. 10am, and don't have a morning snack

Oils for salads:

- Olive or avocado

Oils for frying:

- Butter
- Coconut
- Olive
- Ghee
- Rice Bran

Vegetables

- At least 5–6 types at a time
- Examples: zucchini, cauliflower, beans, carrot, mushroom, sweet potato, beetroot, eggplant, Brussels sprouts, spinach, capsicum

---

**1 fruit serving: 4 small apricots, 1 small apple, 1 cup berries, ½ banana, 1 cup fruit salad, 1 cup grapes, 2 kiwifruit, 2 cups diced honeydew melon, 1 small orange, 1 large nectarine, ½ mango, 2 small mandarins, 1 small pear, 1 large peach, 2 rings fresh pineapple (1cm thick), 3 small plums, ½ cup diced rockmelon, 3 watermelon wedges (1cm thick) or 2 cups diced

*Alternative snack options: ¼ cup mixed nuts, 150 grams yoghurt, carrot sticks or other chopped vegetables, 40 grams (2 slices) cheese, 1 boiled egg, 1 x 210ml glass wine (less than a standard cup)

Chapter Nineteen

My tips for successfully doing Banting/LCHF

- Take it slowly. There is nothing wrong with losing 1 or even half a kilo a month.
- Treat it like a big project, such as renovating a house. Devote time and energy, and plan for it. Don't give up if you have a bad day or a bad week. If halfway through a house renovation you accidentally ordered the wrong tiles for the bathroom, you wouldn't throw your hands up in the air, pull the plug on the whole renovation and live in a half-finished house for the rest of your life. You'd say a few swearwords, send the tiles back and keep going.
- Should you jump straight in or incorporate Banting/LCHF slowly? That's up to you. I think it's better to jump straight in so you aren't constantly making sneaky deals with yourself like, 'I can have sugar in my tea because I've given up wheat.' But if wheat and sugar are too hard for you to exclude at the same time, choose wheat first. Go gluten-free. There are so many

foods that are gluten-free and so many restaurants and take-aways that now serve gluten-free foods. It's easy and you will feel the effects quickly. The cravings for pasta and pastry-type foods will lessen. Don't rely too much on packaged gluten-free foods, though, because they are full of rice flour. Especially gluten-free sausages – I found that out the hard way when we were eating them a lot and I wasn't losing weight. Then I read the packet. When you are ready, go cold turkey on sugar too. All sugars. Honey, maple syrup, corn syrup, artificial sweeteners (they still mess with your head and your appetite for sweet things), fructose, glucose – in fact anything with an 'ose' on the end. And cut down on fruit (down, don't cut it out). This is hard for some people who are extreme fruit lovers, but again, after a few weeks the cravings will lessen. Stick to it. It's difficult at first but it will get easier.

- Discover konjac noodles. You can find these in supermarkets under the label Zero, Miracle Noodles, Slendier noodles and Slim Pasta. They look like rice noodles but are actually made from the root of the konjac plant. So, they are not wheat or rice but a water-soluble vegetable. Referred to as Moyu or Juruo in China, and Konnyaku or Shirataki in Japan, they contain zero net carbohydrates and zero calories. They come in packets and can be stored at room temperature for about a year. They are one of the few exceptions to the don't-eat-food-out-of-a-packet rule. They are translucent and gelatinous, with no flavour of their own, so they easily absorb the flavours of any soup or pasta sauce. To prepare them, rinse them in cold water for about three minutes to get off the fishy-smelling water they come in, then place them in a bowl and pour boiling water over them, leave them to sit for a minute then rinse them again. Easy. And the taste? Okay, I won't pretend they are brilliant and just like pasta, but when you haven't eaten pasta for a year they aren't too bad. You can get them in different styles such as spaghetti, angel hair, rice and lasagne sheets. Make sure you drink lots of water with them and if you react to them in any way stop eating them. Konjac noodles covered with pasta sauce and cheese saved me on many an occasion. I've now also discovered zucchini noodles. We bought a spiraliser and they are so easy to make, and I think they taste even better then konjac noodles. Aprille is a real fan and even makes beetroot noodles, which she fries with a little ginger. So good.

- Exercise gently. Walking is great, as is swimming. You don't have to become a gym junkie – the biggest part of losing weight is diet – but exercise is important. As I said before, exercise makes you feel powerful and strong. Being obese makes you feel weak and hopeless, so anything that gives you confidence is great. I also found that exercise helped connect me to my body again. When I was really overweight my body was just a big lumpy sack I dragged around. I didn't listen to what it needed. I actually never tuned in to it. I ignored all its pleas for help because I didn't know what to do to fix it and because it was all too overwhelming. I had so many body problems I didn't know where to begin, so it was easier to stay in denial. Exercise helps you re-establish the lines of communication with your physical self, which helps you sort out when you are really hungry and when you just want to eat because you are bored/tired/upset/sad/angry. This is crucial.

- If you fall off the wagon, get back on. Straightaway. Not tomorrow, or next week or when some stressful event is over. Don't beat yourself up or go on a binge or throw the whole plan out the window. It happens; it happened to me numerous times. Aprille says that you don't have to eat perfectly all the time, just eat well most of the time. Most of the time does it. Though don't use that as an excuse to eat badly. Every time you eat sugar or wheat the cravings will return and it will take at least a week to restabilise. It's best just to steer clear of them altogether. If you are going to fall off the wagon, go for cheese or nuts.

- Work towards the goal of eating only home-cooked food. I know this is more time-consuming but it's important that you don't rely on packaged foods, even though there is a whole industry now around gluten-free and even Paleo eating. Cavemen didn't eat out of packets and neither should you. Learn to love real food. Vegetables, salads, meat, cheese, nuts, yoghurt. Your body will love you.

Chapter Twenty

How to eat out or order takeaway

- If you love Asian food, I have some bad news for you. Although it's not heavy on wheat, you need to avoid the sauces. Oh, and the rice and rice noodles too. It's also full of sugar and soy (which is wheat-based). Stay away from all Asian restaurants and food stalls. So, no Chinese, Malaysian, Thai or Japanese. Make your favourites at home with wheat-free tamari sauce.
- Indian is great, just don't have the rice. A serve of butter-chicken has saved me at a food court with the kids many times.
- Italian is hard. All that pasta. And don't think gluten-free pizza is okay – the bases are made from soy flour, which is very high carb. You could order the pasta sauce without the pasta – there is nothing wrong with a bowl of carbonara sauce on its own – though I have been on the receiving end of some funny looks doing this.
- German food is great – they do fantastic meats, just avoid the potatoes.

- Vegetarian is also great – so many beautiful choices.
- Good old pub food is the best. They are experts at meat and vegies. Go for the steak and salad/vegie option. Just ask for the steak to have no sauce and the salad to have no dressing.
- Food courts can sometimes be difficult. I was at a food court recently with my son, and of the fifteen or so food options there was only one outlet at which I could eat: the kebab place. And in the kebab place there was only one dish I could order, which I had to modify: kebab meat and salad in a bowl. The salad was sad, wilted lettuce and tomato and the meat was greasy but at least I could eat something and not go hungry. In a food court, look for Indian or a place with lots of salads and vegies or one that does roast meats. Ask for things to be modified or take your own food. Preparation is the key to this way of eating. Being caught out, hungry and eating on the hop is a recipe for disaster.

Chapter Twenty-one

How to cook for yourself and a whole family so you don't have to make two different meals

It's 6 o'clock. You need to cook dinner, then supervise homework, make sure there are clean uniforms for tomorrow, bake a cake for the school fundraiser, then clean the whole house because Auntie Edina is coming over tomorrow and you know she'll comment on the state of the skirting boards, she always does. Oh and you need to make two meals. A Banting/LCHF one for you and something the rest of the family will eat.

But you don't. You can make one family-friendly meal that you modify ever so slightly for yourself.

Here are some ideas . . .

- Spaghetti bolognaise (or any pasta sauce that isn't made with any no-no ingredients): The family has the sauce and pasta, you have the sauce and konjac noodles or zucchini noodles (and lots of cheese!).
- Tacos: The kids have tacos filled with meat, sour cream, lettuce, carrot, grated cheese etc. You have a big lettuce leaf filled with the meat, sour cream, grated cheese, chopped tomato (don't have the tomato sauce in the sachet, it usually has sugar in it).
- Any roast meat and vegies: You skip the potatoes and gravy.
- Hearty winter stew made with sweet potato or pumpkin instead of potato.
- Butter chicken (so good!): Serve with cauliflower couscous. My kids now love it.
- Any fish fried in butter (no flour or breadcrumb coating): Serve with salad or vegies (no potatoes for you).
- Shepherd's pie: Make it with cauliflower mash over the top instead of potato, and lots of cheese over the top too.
- Lamb kofta (just mince lamb on skewers, simple) with a yoghurt dressing.
- Sausages and mash: Make the mash from cauliflower, and make sure the sausages are 100 per cent meat and not made with rice flour.
- Salmon: Serve it baked or fried, no flour coating, and with vegies and/or salad.
- My favourite pasta: Fry chopped onion and bacon, add some vegies, pour in a bottle of passata sauce, bubble away for 30 minutes then add some cream right near the end. You can use tuna instead of bacon but don't use tuna in an olive-oil blend. You have it with konjac or zucchini noodles, and the family has it with pasta.
- Steak/chops with vegies/salad.

- Stir-fry: Any meat with vegies; no Asian sauces in the cooking except tamari or wheat-free soy. Serve with rice for the family, konjac rice or cauliflower rice for you.
- Beef burgers: The burgers are just mince, eggs and onion. Serve with big fluffy sourdough bread rolls for the kids, and you have your burger in lettuce. Add cheese and turn them into cheese-burgers. Add a layer of fried onions and/or mushrooms.

Chapter Twenty-two

How to help your kids cut down on sugar and processed food

I'd love to pretend that I serve the healthiest of foods to my kids, that I've weaned them off sugar and processed foods and we skip happily though a meadow after dinner each night playing guitars and wearing clothes made from curtains. But that's *The Sound of Music* and not the sound in my place. The sound in my place is, 'What's for dessert? I don't like this weird bread. Why did you make muffins again? I want the ones from the shop!'

My kids are far too used to having dessert. I used to equate love with treats and I'm still trying to break that habit. I also used to like treating my kids because I wanted ice-cream or cake, so buying it for them was really just an excuse so I could have some too.

But I am now focused on reducing their sugar and processed foods and feeding them better, although to be clear they are not on a Banting/LCHF diet. We always ate lots of home-cooked meals; it was the snacks and treats that were the problem. Modern advertising has hardwired parents into thinking that kids need to snack all the time. They don't, but I am still trying to get us all out of this thought pattern.

I wish I had a brilliant plan for you about packing school lunches the kids will actually eat, having a healthy snack at hand when they get home from school that they will actually enjoy, and getting them to accept that dessert is a once-in-a-while treat, not an every-night occurrence. I don't. I'm still struggling with all those things.

I guess my advice is to start as early as possible limiting their sugar and processed foods. It gets harder once they are older. I do have the desire and the motivation and am putting in the effort to cut down their sugar and processed-food intake, so this is a start. Any nutritionist would agree that these are important goals to work towards.

Chapter Twenty-three

What I ate (because people keep asking me)

Aprille spends ages getting to know her clients' health history, lifestyle and habits, what they can and can't manage and what they prefer, so this is the plan that she devised for me. It won't suit everyone, because it is based around the foods I love and my sweet spot for weight loss. Everyone will be different.

Breakfast: Half a cup of my homemade cereal and a cup of full-fat milk. My cereal is sesame seeds, flax flakes and chia seeds. If you have a problem with regularity, you won't after several days on this! I don't pre-soak it, because I like it crunchy. And brush your teeth carefully; those chia seeds are little buggers. Once I lost 35 kilos and was having a massive plateau I swapped to two boiled eggs for breakfast to help up my fat intake and reduce my dairy intake then I swapped back to the seeds as I needed the regularity but I changed the milk to Greek yoghurt.

Lunch: Last night's dinner.

Dinner: Protein (usually meat, fish or eggs) and vegies covered in butter.

Dessert: 150 grams made up of double cream and Greek yoghurt, plus a scattering of berries. I eventually cut out the berries because they were too sweet for me and triggered my cravings, and then I cut out the cream and yoghurt because I was cutting down on my dairy so I now have no dessert at all.

Snacks: One handful of macadamias and one orange.

Drinks: Water, lots of water. Aprille got me on to soda water, which I now love. It's great when you are tempted to snack. Aprille taught me about the three types of hunger – brain hunger (cravings), mouth hunger (boredom and habit) and body hunger (real physical hunger). I realised that most of my hunger was the mouth type, which soda water helps abate. I also started drinking dandelion coffee. As Aprille got me off coffee and tea to improve my sleep, which it did, this was my alternative. I have two cups a day with full-cream milk, and I changed this to one with milk and one with double cream when I had my really big plateau.

Supplements: Vitamin D, iron and magnesium (because I was low in all three). Get yourself tested before adding iron and magnesium and vitamin D to your diet, but you will probably find you are low in D, especially if like me you work in an office.

That was it. If I was starving I would have a slice of cheese with avocado on it. I defy anyone to be hungry after that. It is a real hunger buster.

Chapter Twenty-four

The first few weeks

You have been on a vicious cycle that has gone round and round while your weight has gone up and up.

We need to break that cycle.

You do this first by eating foods that don't raise your insulin, and to do that you have to ignore those nasty constant cravings for instant-energy high-carb foods. And that's tough. In the first few days, even weeks, your body will scream (even more than it used to) for pasta and bread and sweets. Ignore it. Tell yourself that these foods don't make the cravings go away, that they always come back. Tell yourself that you are breaking this cycle and the cravings will lesson or even go away completely if you stick to the plan. Tell yourself to just keep going.

After a few days or weeks of no insulin spikes, your body will get used to drawing on your supplies of fat and will stop freaking out. The cravings will lessen, and you will have more energy because your cells will have a steady supply of energy. Your brain will also function better, you will be clearer and won't have your usual 3pm brain crash every day.

This can happen quickly for some, more slowly for others. That's why giving in and eating a cupcake puts you back on the vicious cycle and means you have to break it all over again and deal with the high level of cravings again too.

Tell yourself that the cupcake actually feeds and perpetuates the cravings rather than stops them.

Be gentle on yourself. This is a big transition your body is making. You are transitioning from the up–down, spike–crash of muscles, tissues and brain starving for energy because your body keeps stashing the incoming energy away in your fat cells, to a steady supply of fuel that is calming and healing.

Tell yourself over and over that you are working towards a peaceful, calm freedom that is worth it.

Don't worry about portion size during this phase. Eat lots of fat. Eat handfuls of nuts and chunks of cheese and avocado. And don't worry if the scale doesn't shift much or at all. Once things calm down and you're not screaming for carbs constantly, you can focus on how much you eat.

Here are some other things you may encounter.

Fatigue

Your body is still in old mode. Your muscles, tissues and brain are deprived of fuel and tell your body to be as sedentary as possible to preserve energy. In the past you would have fixed this by eating a tsunami of easily digested energy in the form of highly processed carbs. This was my 3pm dim-sims-and-pine-apple-donut fix. I would eat for short-term energy and then my energy would crash and I would eat for short-term energy again, and so on it went. Keep going, knowing this will pass and you will have more, steadier energy in the future than you have ever had.

Bad breath

Your body is transitioning from burning glucose to burning those fatty acids or ketones. It's the ketones you (and others, I'm afraid) can smell on your breath. That's good. Keep going. This is a good sign and it will fade. Drinks lots of water to help rid yourself of this early symptom.

Headache

For the first three or so days you may have a headache – just like if you stopped smoking or drinking alcohol suddenly you would get withdrawal headaches. It will pass. This is normal. Carbs are very addictive. Lots of water will help this too. It's another reason to not eat that cupcake, because you will have to go through the withdrawal headache again when you get back on the program.

Muscle cramps

Carbs retain water, so your body will be dumping excess fluid in the first few weeks. You will look less puffy, which is great, but you will also lose salt and other minerals and this is what causes the cramps. Put good-quality sea salt or rock salt on your food and increase your intake of green leafy vegies to replace the magnesium and potassium you are losing.

Constipation

Some people suffer from constipation while doing Banting/LCHF. I actually found the opposite and it cured my life-long constipation. But if it does block you up, try upping your water intake and increase your fibrous vegetables such as cabbage and Brussels sprouts. If your vegetable intake is already high, then try Professor Noakes's cure – add 2 tablespoons of psyllium husks to your daily diet. Aprille suggests a teaspoon of coconut oil daily and as a last measure taking a stool softener to get things moving.

Money drain

Something that will feel lighter is your wallet. This way of eating isn't cheap, because you are eating high-quality foods. Pasta and bread are cheap. A beautiful steak ribbed with fat and served with a blue-cheese sauce is not cheap. That sucks. You will be eating less overall and also snacking less, so there are money-saving advantages over time. And you will have more energy and will get sick less often, which also helps the finances. Plus, you will be eating your leftovers rather than letting them become a mould-growing science experiment in the back of the fridge. You won't be eating on the hop anymore, you will be organised and have some nuts and water on you at all times. Vegetables are also very cost effective and will be the main thing you eat. But if money is holding you back from eating this way, go for cheap mince rather than steak. The cheaper the better. Expensive five-star mince is lean, the cheap stuff is full of beautiful fat. You will also be doing a lot more cooking. Pre-prepared meals such as satay sticks are expensive compared to making them yourself. Keep going. Prioritise your health. Don't have a holiday this year. Or a new winter coat. And if you are really struggling financially, you have my heart-felt sympathy. Being poor sucks. I've been there for years with my part-time jobs and constant pile of bills I didn't know how to pay. It's depressing and encourages you to eat cheap foods such as chocolate, chips and pizza.

Here's some advice for doing Banting on a budget:

- Learn to really love eggs.
- Don't bake LCHF versions of cakes and muffins. Almond flour and flaxseed meal are expensive. Stick to eating the basics – eggs/meat/fish and vegies.
- Buy butter and other staples in bulk.
- Bake food rather than fry. Coconut oil is expensive and you use a lot when frying.
- Eat less-popular parts of animals. Offal, kidneys, cheeks, shoulders are all cheaper cuts that are just as good. (Okay, I can't do offal but I do eat kidneys.)
- Don't go organic. Strange advice, I know, but it is better to eat LCHF with conventionally raised meat and vegies than to not eat LCHF at all. Organic can wait until your financial position improves.
- Eat seasonally. What's plentiful and hasn't been shipped from the other side of the world is usually cheaper.

Time poor

This kind of poor can be equally depressing. You work, you study, you serve on committees, you devote time to your kids' school or to a local charity and you run and run and run. You wake up early and the running begins. Isn't it easier just to shove some packets in the kids' lunch boxes and have take-away for dinner? Yes, it is easier but it is even easier to be hectic when you feel good and fit into your clothes and into the car. The steering wheel of my car used to press against my stomach, which was no fun when doing the constant drop-offs and pick-ups that parents do, and probably not very safe either. 'Hello, officer, sorry I ran over the kerb, I couldn't turn the steering wheel because of my gigantic stomach.' Not a conversation I ever had to have, luckily, and not one you want to have either. So, make the time. Order online from the supermarket once a week and get it delivered to your door instead of doing the big weekly shop. Cook in bulk and freeze some for later. Prioritise your health. Learn to say no. Do Banting with a friend and cook in bulk together once a week. Be creative. Let the house get messy, or in my case, messier. Look at your priorities. Someone else can chair the school-toilet-redecorating committee, you're too busy redecorating yourself.

Chapter Twenty-five

Help! I've stopped losing weight!

Welcome to Plateau Land. I'm a long-time resident of Plateau Land, so let me show you around. It's very flat here. And still. The view is identical in every direction you look. Oh, and we have a strange phenomenon: no matter how often you weigh yourself, the scales never change. In Plateau Land no matter how hard you work, how many laps you swim or how many heavy weights you lift, the scales don't budge. And it feels like you will be here forever.

What can you do? Sometimes you need to just accept it and enjoy your stay. You've made a lot of changes and dropped a lot of weight, so just cruise and enjoy the success you have had so far in the knowledge that your body will start losing weight again when it is ready. Don't stress, and whatever you do don't give up and undo all your good work. But if you suspect there may be something causing your extended vacation in Plateau Land, especially if your time there is going on far too long – say, more than two weeks – here are my tips for getting a speedy exit visa out of there!

Too many sneaky carbs

It was the gluten-free sausages that caused one of my many plateaus. They're gluten-free! They're just meat, right? Wrong. I read the packet, something I should have done when I started buying them. They were chockful of rice flour. Check the labels and go back to doing an online food diary so you can see exactly how many carbs you are eating. You may be surprised at how many carbs are sneaking in. Lots of fruit can be a real culprit here.

Too many calories

Remember that you want your body to dip into its fat stores and to do that you need to eat less than your body needs each day. If you have lost a lot of weight your RDI may now be lower. Go back and work it out again and also go back to the online food diary. You may need to look at your portion sizes and cut them back.

Not enough fat?

When I am really hungry I have a small slice of cheese with avocado on it. Upping my good fats intake made a huge difference to my hunger, dropping it right down so I ate much less. Try it. And if you don't like avocado try a spoonful of coconut oil. And if you can't stomach that try the Paleo bullet coffee occasionally – black coffee with butter and coconut oil whisked in. Not to my taste but many people swear by it.

Too many nuts

Oh yes, that handful of nuts can easily become two or three handfuls. Nuts can be your undoing.

Too much snacking

Snacking all day long will not teach your body to dip into its fat stores. Try to stick to your main meals and one or two snacks. This is not a grazing diet.

Not enough salt

This may surprise you. When you were eating a lot of processed food you were probably eating too much salt. Now that everything is home cooked you possibly aren't getting enough. Try adding some good-quality sea salt or rock salt to your food (no, not your yoghurt) and see if that helps your hunger levels to go down and for you to feel better overall.

Too much milk and yoghurt

Lactose is the milk sugar that makes milk and yoghurt taste sweet. Be careful of how much milk and yoghurt you consume. Aged dairy such as hard cheese is better. Plus, milk is also high in protein, which can be problematic. This doesn't apply to butter.

Too much protein

Is that steak on your plate taking up the whole plate? Is it hanging over the edges? It shouldn't be, unless you are eating off a really small plate. Remember that this isn't a high-protein diet and that protein still spikes your insulin. Cut back on your protein and increase your vegetables and see if that helps.

Are you expecting to lose too much, too quickly?

Maybe you are having a plateau or maybe you are confusing slow steady weight loss of a kilo a month with a plateau. Maybe you need to lower your expectations. You *will* get lean and you *will* stay lean and it doesn't have to happen by tomorrow. Slower is better for some people and more sustainable. Don't worry about going slowly.

Doing too much exercise or not enough?

This is a damned-if-you-do-and-damned-if-you-don't scenario. Exercise will definitely help your weight loss but too much will hinder it, especially long sessions of low-impact exercise such as jogging for hours. It will make you really hungry and can cause you to overeat. Three to four times per week of high-intensity short-duration exercise is best for weight loss.

Should you try fasting?

At one stage, to shift a plateau, Aprille had me fast till midday each day then eat lunch, a snack, then dinner, then fast again. This was a sixteen-hour fast every day and it really helped. I didn't find it sustainable long term but there is a lot of good research about the benefits of fasts. Another reason to stop eating at 8pm and not eat until breakfast at around 7am – that is an eleven-hour fast right there every day and very doable.

Are you taking vitamin D?

It has been known for a while that low levels of vitamin D are linked to obesity, but a new study at the University of Milan has shown that taking vitamin D can actually help you lose weight. The study recruited 400 obese and overweight people and divided them into three groups. The first took no vitamin D, the second took 25,000 IU per month and the third took a whopping 100,000 IU per month. All 400 were then put on the same low-calorie diet. After six months, those who took 100,000 IU per month achieved the highest average weight loss of 11.9 pounds. The 25,000 IU group lost an average of 8.4 pounds, while those who took nothing lost 2.6 pounds. The researchers concluded that, 'All people affected by obesity should have their levels of vitamin D tested to see if they are deficient, and if so, begin taking supplements.' So please, get your levels checked and supplement with vitamin D if you are low.

Apple cider vinegar?

I've just started taking a tablespoon of apple cider vinegar in soda water every night. It can help control blood sugar levels and prevent spikes. Aprille is a big fan of apple cider vinegar.

Going for a walk after dinner?

This was mentioned to me as a way to get my stomach to release leptin, the hormone that tells the brain that the stomach is full and to stop eating. Those of us who have overeaten for years may find that our stomach is stretched and not as good at recognising that it is full. Gentle movement like a walk helps the lining of the stomach recognise fullness and therefore to signal the brain with the release of leptin. It is also a good habit that enforces that dinner is over and you are progressing into the non-eating part of the evening. It's also a nice thing to do to release the stresses of the day and wind down into the evening, either out on your own or with your partner and kids. It can be just a twenty-minute walk around the block. It doesn't have to be the 800-kilometre Camino de Santiago, the pilgrim's walk through northwestern Spain. My sisters-in-law Glenda and Lyn did this last year and came back with great stories and buns of steel. You don't need buns of steel, you just need twenty minutes and a safe route.

Chapter Twenty-six

The last few kilos

Welcome to the hard part. Yes, I know, that's unfair. You've done so much and come so far. This should be smooth sailing, but it isn't.

As Aprille says, little changes make a huge difference at the start because you have been eating so badly and not exercising (or at least I wasn't much), but now small mistakes make a huge difference.

I actually put weight on during this last phase, something that had only happened once in my whole journey, when I had been snacking on cupcakes. There wasn't a cupcake in a ten-mile radius of me at this point and I was putting weight on! I was sticking 100 per cent to this way of eating but I was just eating too much. Damn those sneaky nuts.

Here are some tips:

• Keep going, don't give up and undo all your hard work.

- Do you need to revise your final weight? Is it the weight you were at when you were twenty? Is it unrealistic to be that weight again?
- Can you cut back on portion sizes?
- Can you go lower carb?
- Do you need to go back to doing an online food diary to check your carb, protein and calorie levels?
- Can you eat more fat, even just temporarily?
- Is this just a plateau? Look back at the 'Help! I've stopped losing weight!' section to try some of the plateau-breaking tips.
- How's your exercise? Are you doing enough? Can you fit in three or four high-intensity short-duration workouts per week? Or are you doing too much and making yourself really hungry?

The main thing here is to *keep going*. I know someone who lost 50 kilos of a 60-kilo goal and then plateaued for a whole year; she gave up on losing more and put 10 kilos back on straightaway. Luckily she stopped herself before she put it all back on again, but now she regrets it because she has to work hard to get those 10 kilos off. If she had just been happy with losing 50 kilos and let that plateau take as long as it needed she could have stayed at that point until her body was ready to drop more weight again. Plateaus do your head in, they really do.

Be patient, with the scales and with yourself.

You'll get there. And remember, you are eating this way as much for good health as for weight loss. Your insides are loving you.

Love yourself back and take your time.

Chapter Twenty-seven

Now that I've lost all the weight, what can I eat?

You really want me to say that you can eat anything you like, don't you? Sorry, I am not going to say that, but you don't have to watch your portion sizes as much. Just eat when you're hungry and stop when you're full. And keep eating LCHF. It's so good for your health, your hormones, your blood sugar, your whole body.

And remember that eating a big piece of chocolate cake will just spike your insulin and bring all those nasty cravings back again and you will then have two pieces or three and before you know it you've eaten badly for a week and put five kilos back on.

Aprille suggests that once you reach your desired goal you give yourself a 2-kilo window and still weigh yourself every morning. If you ever go higher than that 2-kilo limit you need to go back to being strict until you are at your goal weight. It's normal for weight to fluctuate, but you need to make sure you stay in your 2-kilo comfort zone.

You also need to pat yourself on the back. Big time. You've made it. You are in control now, not your cravings. You are awesome. Say it with me . . . awesome . . . in the true sense of the word: worthy of awe.

Or go have two squares of dark chocolate (70 per cent cocoa or above). You deserve it, and now you can have it. But no more than two squares. I'm watching you.

Chapter Twenty-eight

A final word about the diet industry

Dieting, over time, makes you fat. And by dieting I mean cutting calories.

Just in case you were tempted to give up on LCHF and go back to the conventional approach to weight loss, let me spell this out for you. Going on a diet has a very good chance of making you fatter in the long term. Going on many diets over many years has a very good chance of making you very fat. And this is independent of your genetics, age or gender.

Not only are you not a lazy glutton, but the approach the weight-loss industry has been telling you to take has actually made the problem worse. In fact, all those diets you've gone on since you had a tiny weight problem in your youth have actually contributed significantly to the major weight problem you might have now.

And here's the proof. This weight-increasing effect of dieting was examined in a Finnish study on more than 2000 sets of twins.

The ones who had dieted, even just once, were two to three times more likely to become overweight compared to their non-dieting twin. Two to three times more likely! And even more alarming, the more times a twin dieted the higher the risk of becoming overweight became.

This isn't new news. There have been other studies confirming this fact dating back sixty years. A group of UCLA researchers reviewed thirty-one long-term studies on the effectiveness of dieting and concluded that dieting is a consistent predictor of weight gain – with up to two-thirds of the people regaining more weight than they lost.

So, why hasn't the weight-loss industry completely changed its approach? Because failed dieters are great return clients.

I can't say this enough – dieting is a short-term fix that has long-term consequences. Any diet company can trot out a successful client and say, 'Ta da! It works.' But it doesn't work for the majority of clients and it certainly doesn't work in the long term. How many celebrities who have done Jenny Craig have put all the weight back on again and then some? Even *The Biggest Loser* TV show has a pretty poor long-term outlook. I used to love this show. I watched it slavishly, hoping its weight-loss magic would infuse itself through the nano rays of television into me as I watched all the contestants run up and down sand dunes while I ate Tim Tams on the couch.

A new research study (you know I love my studies) just published in the *Obesity Journal* tracked fourteen contestants from the eighth American season of *The Biggest Loser* for six years post filming. Thirteen out of the fourteen former contestants put back on large amounts of weight in that time; four actually weighed more than they did at the beginning of the show. This doesn't surprise me. The last time I watched the Australian version of

The Biggest Loser the contestants were sitting around enjoying a snack of diet yoghurt after a heavy workout, their tubs prominently held up so the camera could linger on the label, which happened to belong to a sponsor of the show. Diet yoghurts contain around 16 grams of sugar. That's four teaspoons. Diet yoghurts are just dairy-flavoured sugar in a tub. Crash diets, eating processed foods and exercise programs that aren't sustainable in the real world doom these contestants to failure. And this American study just proved it.

And what's worse than the weight-loss industry hiding this information from you, they are actively targeting people who speak out against it.

Emeritus Professor Tim Noakes, the South African Banting expert, is fighting for his career after been charged with unprofessional conduct by The Health Professions Council of South Africa. A mother had asked Professor Noakes via Twitter how the Banting diet could be applied to her situation: she was breastfeeding. Her Tweet read: '@ProfTimNoakes is LCHF eating ok for breastfeeding mums? Worried about all the dairy + cauliflower = wind for babies??'

Professor Noakes responded: 'Baby doesn't eat the dairy and cauliflower. Just very healthy high-fat breast milk. Key is to wean baby onto LCHF.'

The Association for Dietetics in South Africa (ADSA) is driving this attack. They made an official complaint about this Tweet, which led to the charge. Professor Noakes could lose his medical licence over this. But he has stood by his advice, saying that babies should ideally be breastfed and then weaned onto real, unprocessed foods such as meat, vegetables and dairy as opposed to manufactured baby cereal that contains sugar. I am watching this trial with great interest.

Don't doubt for a second that the processed-food industry doesn't want you to try Banting either. A recent investigation has shown that in 2015 the ADSA was sponsored by companies such as Huletts Sugar, Kellogg's, Woolworths, Unilever and Parmalat, which all make their very large profits from us eating processed foods. In fact, Kellogg's, one of the companies that started the world eating sugary wheat cereal for breakfast instead of eggs, is the ADSA's gold sponsor and has staff on its executive committee. And Coca-Cola has sponsored the ADSA's nutrition education events. Coca-Cola has even set up an entire organisation to make sure you don't get the anti-sugar message. It's called The Beverage Institute for Health and Wellness. Its main role is as 'A Resource for Health Professionals on the Science of Beverages, Hydration & Active Healthy Living', which translates as: *If you exercise more and eat less you will be healthy.* i.e. *The problem is that you are a lazy glutton and has nothing to do with the sugar industry.*

Your average nutritionist or dietician doesn't want you to try this either. Partly because they are wedded to the 'everything in moderation' model that you and I know doesn't work. But also, I suspect, because deep down in their hearts they can't embrace a system that doesn't blame fat people for the way they are. Lots of nutritionists, with the exception of Aprille, are born thin and stay naturally thin and believe we fat people are just lazy gluttons and that this is our real problem. That we lack willpower, the kind of willpower that they must have in spades because they are thin. They've never been called disgusting. They've never had every cell in their body screaming for food. They have no idea what it's really like to battle these cravings. They just think we should be like them and eat a little bit of everything. Well, that model has worked brilliantly for us so far, hasn't it? That model is doing a great job of defeating the obesity epidemic that is sweeping the developed world, ruining our health and draining our health-system budgets.

I can't say this enough: You are not a lazy glutton. You never were. It's not you. It's them. Stop listening to them and start taking control of your own body, your own life and your own health.

I have, and I really hope that you will join me.

Chapter Twenty-nine

FAQs

Is this diet Atkins?
No, Atkins is higher protein than Banting/LCHF. This is high-fat, moderate-protein, low-carb. Atkins is low-carb high-protein.

Is it Paleo?
No. Paleo is low in carbs, but not as low as this. Paleo cuts out cereals but it also cuts out dairy, which we love.

Are you anti fat people?
No! I was overweight off and on (but more on) for thirty-four years. I am anti how bad being overweight is for your health.

What if I am diabetic?
You need to check with your doctor before changing your diet, because it may require you to adjust your medication.

What if I already have heart disease?
Again, check with your doctor before changing your diet, because you may need to adjust your medication.

But doesn't eating fat make you fat and clog your arteries?
No. There isn't a scientific study that has actually proven a link between eating saturated fat and artery clogging, otherwise known as atherosclerosis, which leads to heart attacks. Studies have certainly shown a link between being overweight or obese and atherosclerosis, and because it was once believed that fat makes you fat the leap was then made that eating fat causes heart attacks. Insulin resistance is a risk factor in heart disease and you get that by eating a high level of carbs, not fat. Another risk factor for heart disease is having a diet high in trans-fats and Omega 6, and Banting/LCHF does not include these fats in its good-fats list.

How often should I weigh myself?
Every morning, first thing, is best. Your weight will fluctuate day to day but weighing yourself every day keeps you on track better than once a week. If you are obsessing about that red flashing number, though, then once a week is fine.

What if I'm a vegetarian?
You can do Banting/LCHF as a vegetarian. You just have to watch that you don't eat too many vegetables that are high in carbohydrates, and avoid lentils and soy products. Eggs, dairy and nuts will be your go-to fat and protein source. If you can add fish, even better.

Won't I get cancer if I eat lots of red meat?
A lot of the studies that showed a higher risk of cancer for meat eaters versus vegetarians didn't factor in that the meat eaters

surveyed also smoked, ate junk food and didn't exercise. There is a slightly higher risk for red-meat eaters of getting colon cancer and this needs to be taken seriously. Don't make red meat your daily staple. Chicken and fish don't come with this slightly higher risk, so mix your diet up. Also, try not to blacken red meat when you cook it, because this has been shown to produce dangerous substances that could harm your health. But remember that it is only a slightly higher risk and by being overweight or obese you are increasing your risk of getting all cancers by a much higher factor. Always fry meat of any kind in good oils that don't go rancid. Remember, this isn't a high-protein diet, it is a high-vegetable diet. If you are eating red meat at every meal you are doing LCHF wrong.

What if I don't like eating fat?

We've been told for years to cut the fat off meat and bacon, and for some people it is hard to go back to eating it. But remember, there are many types of food that contain good fats: eggs, dairy, butter, avocados, coconut oil, olive oil, ghee, lard, duck fat, macadamia nuts and macadamia oil. Experiment with what works for you.

What if I hate eggs for breakfast (or at any other time of the day)?

Then don't eat them. Don't eat anything you don't like. Just go with meat, cheese, dairy, nuts and vegies. Fried saganaki cheese and wilted spinach for breakfast is delicious.

I have a real sweet tooth. Surely a bit of honey is okay?

No, it isn't. You need to lose that sweet tooth completely, and it will go away if you cut out all sugars.

Is there anyone who should not do Banting/LCHF?
Yes, anyone who has a medical issue and hasn't discussed Banting/ LCHF with their doctor. And nor should anyone who is naturally very lean and does a lot of regular exercise. But especially anyone who, after regular cholesterol checks, finds that Banting/LCHF increases their total and LDL cholesterol.

Can I have a cheat day?
Of course you can. I can't stop you. You can have a cheat day, a cheat week or even a cheat month. But you will pay the consequences and will go back to all those cravings. Is it worth it? This isn't a 'diet' that should make you feel the need to cheat. This is a way of life that leads to freedom. Why would you cheat yourself out of that?

Chapter Thirty

Resources for lots more info

There are many eminent scientists and medical authorities who are championing Banting/LCHF as a way to fight the obesity and type-2 diabetes epidemic, so I urge you to check out their wisdom, research and protocols for living this liberating lifestyle.

Professor Tim Noakes www.realmealrevolution.com
Books: *The Real Meal Revolution, Super Food for Superchildren*

Dr Andreas Eenfeldt, the Swedish physician and LCHF expert
www.dietdoctor.com

Dr Jason Fung, a Toronto-based nephrologist (a kidney expert)
www.intensivedietarymanagement.com
Book: *The Obesity Code: Unlocking the Secrets of Weight Loss*

Dr Joseph Michael Mercola, an American osteopathic physician
www.mercola.com

Dr David Perlmutter, an American neurologist
www.drperlmutter.com
Book: *Grain Brain*

Dr Aseem Malhotra, a British cardiologist
www.doctoraseem.com

Dr Zoë Harcombe, a British obesity researcher
www.zoeharcombe.com

Gary Taubes, an American science writer
Books: *Good Calories, Bad Calories* (for those with a scientific or medical background)

Why We Get Fat (the same information for the lay person)

Nina Teicholz, an American science journalist
Book: *The Big, Fat Surprise: Why Butter, Meat & Cheese Belong in a Healthy Diet*

Dr Sandra Aamodt, an American neuroscientist
www.sandraaamodt.com
TED talk: *Why Dieting Doesn't Usually Work*

Cereal Killers I and *Cereal Killers II*, the two cult documentaries about Banting/LCHF www.cerealkillersmovie.com

That Sugar Film, an Australian film about sugar addiction
www.thatsugarfilm.com

David Gillespie, Australian anti-sugar campaigner
www.davidgillespie.org

And of course, do check out Aprille's website
www.aprillemcmahonnutritionist.com.au

And Mischa's website www.boxingcentral.com.au

Also, join my Facebook page Death by Dim Sim where I post lots of scientific updates, recipes, advice and tips and where you can get support and encouragement from me and the Death by Dim Sim community.

Acknowledgements

The day I found out this book was going to be published by Penguin Random House I bought a big cake to take home after work. A caramel and banana frosted monster as big as a car wheel. Not that I was going to eat any of it. I was going to watch my family eat it. Over several nights, I hoped. When I lugged it off the train I wondered why I had bought such a big cake. Because this was a very big moment, I realised. I had wanted to be a published author since I was ten. Two dreams – being released from my prison of fat and becoming an author – had come true at the same time. It was momentous. Life was never going to be the same again.

I then decided I wanted to cut the cake with lots of the people I loved and who had supported both my writing and my weight loss. It was 6.30pm on a Tuesday night. Would anyone be around?

I quickly sent a group text message to all our friends who lived locally. We'd met each other through our children's primary school. We minded each other's kids, we went on holidays together, some of us had even formed a book group. We had been there for each other through many ups and downs. In the text message I said my book was being published and to come over at 8pm for cake and champagne. It was a school night and was well into the busy holiday season. Would anyone come?

Text messages started arriving back. Sulari was busy, as was Chris, Imogen and Terri. They all sent me excited messages but couldn't pop over that night for different reasons (a restless baby, kids' sports commitments, husbands working late). The giant cake started to feel very heavy and a bit silly. Then more messages arrived. Aprille was coming and so was Mim. David and Denise were coming too, as were Caroline and Chris, Andrea and David, Kylie and Anita plus a bunch of their kids.

When everyone arrived I lifted up a bottle of champagne, pointed it at the roof and eased the cork off. It shot out with a loud bang. Someone called out 'Plasterer!' as it bounced off the ceiling.

I poured everyone a glass, and a glass of soda water for myself. I cut everyone but me a piece of cake. You can't have your cake and eat it too, but you can watch people you love eat it, which is just as good.

Russell wrapped an arm around me. 'I'm so happy for you,' he said. Then he paused and looked puzzled. 'But I still don't understand why anyone would want to read a book about us. We're so ordinary.'

I looked around our ordinary house, at our ordinary (eccentric) pets, our ordinary (amazing, supportive) friends, our ordinary (funny, smart, healthy) kids and then back at my ordinary (loving, kind, handsome, talented) husband.

'Ordinary rocks,' I told him. And it does. Thank you, friends and family, for all your support. I couldn't have done it without you.

A few individual thank yous I especially want to make. Thank you to all my tutors and fellow students in the RMIT Professional Writing and Editing program, especially my co-students and friends The Writerley Ladies. To Writers Victoria and its amazing staff, volunteers and members for all their support. To Varuna and Patti Miller for getting me started on this book. Thank you also to the ACT Writers Centre's Hardcopy program and the writers in the program with whom I shared that extraordinary journey, plus Nigel Hardcastle and Mary Cunnane who guided us. To my agent Jacinta Di Mase and to everyone at Penguin Random House, especially Meredith Curnow for her early support, and to Sophie Ambrose for her extraordinary structural edit and wisdom. Plus, a huge thank you to copyeditor Claire de Medici and to my writing group, the Line Tamers, Shivaun Plozza, Rosey Chang, Marie Davies and Cathy Hainstock. I couldn't have written this book without all of these generous and inspiring champions in my corner. Also thank you to Katie Miles for digging out her 21st birthday photos from her attic, and to Dr Debbie Herbst, GP, for her help with the science section. And lastly to my trainer Mischa Merz and my nutritionist Aprille McMahon for both putting up with me and having faith in me.

PQ00492073